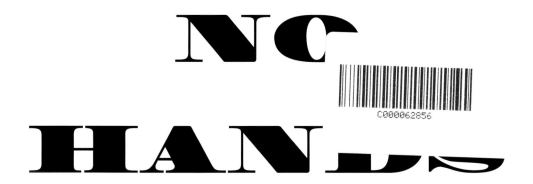

NO HANDS

Chair Massage

—⇒∘⇐—

Conversations between Tonto and the Lone Ranger

Gerry Pyves
David Woodhouse

Shi'Zen Publications

Published by Shi'Zen Publications
PO Box 57, Hebden Bridge, W.Yorks, HX7 6WW
www.shizen.co.uk

Drawings by John Coombes
Photography by Stephen Lord
Illustrations and cover by Sean Creagh
Proofing by Angie Cairns
Lay-out and design by Mike Barrett
Printed in Great Britain by The Charlesworth Group, Huddersfield
ISBN 0-9539074-1-4

No Hands Chair Massage is the second book in the NO HANDS trilogy.
The first is The Principles and Practice of No Hands Massage by Gerry Pyves also published by Shi'Zen Publications

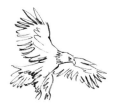

DEDICATION

This book is dedicated to all massage practitioners, wherever you may be.

Gerry would also like to make a personal dedication to the memory of his father, Peter Pyves, who died whilst the book was being written.

"You probably would not have made sense of a single word of it had you lived to read it - but nobody would have been more proud of its achievement than you. God bless you, Dad."

ACKNOWLEDEGMENTS

So many people are involved in the production of a book like this.

The authors would firstly like to thank Geraldine Scott. Your unstinting support of us has been nothing short of magnificent. You were present at those first tentative beginnings, and it was you who suggested "Why not write it like a conversation?" Little did you know what you had set in motion! Your painstaking reading and re-reading of every word of this text as it neared completion was heroic. Not once did you complain at the numerous late-night telephone editing sessions. For this the authors have awarded you the title of honorary midwife to the birth of this book!

The authors would like to thank the many practitioners and trainers who have also contributed to the ideas and the theories here, particularly all the trainers and students whom we are both privileged to work with on a regular basis – you all know who you are. In particular we would like to say a big "thank you" for the written contributions of the four gifted practitioners who are such an important part of this book: Ruari Martin, Judy Midgely, Peter Mackereth and Gwynneth Campbell. You are all doing so much to support the work of practitioners everywhere.

The authors would also like to acknowledge all the practitioners who attended those first wildly creative NO HANDS Chair Massage workshops in which we invented over 80 new Chair strokes, some of which, thankfully, will never see the light of day again!

We would also like to acknowledge the outstanding talents of the whole Shi'Zen publishing team: Angie Cairns for your sensitive and expert proofing; Sean Creagh, for your beautiful map and illustrations - and your inspired contributions to the whole Wild West feel to this book including your magnificent cover; Stephen Lord for your stunning photography; and finally we would like to acknowledge Mike Barrett for your tasteful lay-out - as ever, your creativity is a sheer delight to witness. The humour and pleasantness with which you carried out your respective crafts are as much a delight to us as the sheer quality of your work.

The authors would also like to acknowledge John Coombes – for your unbelievable talent in drawing and painting the human body. It would be worth writing a bodywork book a year, just for an excuse to spend more time in your magnificent Millbank studio!

And finally, we would both like to acknowledge our long-suffering families. Without your reminders that there is more to life than massage, we would have both floated off into the land of nonsense years ago. Your loving support is evident in every page of this book.

CONTENTS

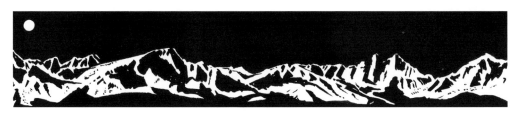

IN CELEBRATION OF
THE CHAIR

We are currently witnessing the greatest explosion of touch in the public arena ever known to modern man and woman.

Yes we are,

　　Honestly!

　　　　And **Chair Massage** is doing it,

　　　　　　all over the world

And Massage Practitioners are doing it.

　　All over the world

　　　　you are doing it,

　　　　　　or thinking about doing it if you are reading this:

Spreading your own brand of peace through your touch ...

How much war would there be if all the politicians took in a Chair Massage on the way to their parliaments and their meeting places ...

and the practitioner simply nurtured them into silence and stillness with the irresistible potency of total focus, powerful posture

and a lifetime's dedication to healing?

So that our politicians could once again feel the loving hands of God caress their bruised and battered egos and psyches

kneading them back into wholeness ...

And when they get to their meetings, walking on air, listening to the birds, seeing the beauty of the sun upon their parliament buildings, in short, when they are reminded of their own divinity, no less

- where they had originally feared to meet hostility and had planned to survive with posture and threats and thereby risk the lives and welfare of whole populations of gentle families with honest hard-working parents, instead, when they look across their meeting tables

all they see are the tear-stained eyes of God looking back at them, *beseeching* them to build peace and understanding,

and instead of sitting opposite them at the table in confrontational mode,

our dedicated politicians walk around the table and sit beside their erstwhile opponents and simply ask

"What can we do to help you?",

thereby setting in motion a whole chain of events

that brings down armaments factories

and leaves the bellicose warmongers without an audience,

simply because

everyone is too busy queuing up

for that Chair Massage in the market place ...

So you see, there is no greater mission on the planet right now

than

the mission of touch ...

Today you will meet practitioners with virtually no income to their name actually *paying* to work in public places!

Practitioners who were themselves touched by this exploding, cascading, absolutely unstoppable wave of touch wellness and touch healing that is Chair Massage *and actually became part of the wave itself ...*

and Chair Massage really does it, with

its unique combination of the *visually fascinating* with the *powerfully therapeutic ...*

All over the world in malls and airports, in conference centres and exhibition halls, in corporate offices and government buildings we can see it:

the power that is Chair Massage:

touch reaching out to people who would never contemplate taking their clothes off in a room alone with a stranger.

People opening their wallets to pay for a bodywork session in a public place – people who would never contemplate paying the fees that practitioners charge for their powerful therapeutic work in private clinics and treatment rooms –

and practitioners are doing it,

practitioners who stand in the marketplace banging their drums and singing their crazy mad songs of touch salvation,

because that is what is happening, and

in all the world,

only massage practitioners are doing it:

greeting, touching and saying goodbye to hundreds of grateful people who go on their way ...

forgetting their shopping lists and wandering aimlessly through the malls seeing only the beauty of humanity,

Momentarily forgetting to be at war in their offices, and inadvertently buying flowers instead of penning vicious memos ...

all of them

      transformed, and

          just for a moment

              remembering something ...

                    something numinous,

                        something beyond

                            simply hearing:

echoes ... of the hand of God.

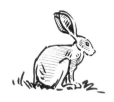

About Bodywork, Chair Massage and a Book that just wouldn't get written, until...

A S DAVID AND I STARTED SENDING THE CONVERSATIONAL MES-
SAGES to each other that formed the basis of this book, we instinctively
started addressing each other as Tonto and Kemo-Sabe. At first, this was
in jest. A bit of fun ...

As time went on, however, we both began to realise that the Lone Ranger and
Tonto were wonderful archetypes of our modern age, archetypes of integrity,
honesty and collaboration. In Tonto we have an archetype of spiritual depth
and skilful awareness of the earth. In the Lone Ranger we have an archetype of
courage and integrity.

One day, early into this collaboration, David and I were discussing yet again
how to present our ideas for a book that had got a bit stuck, and we just looked
up at each other and said, "Why not write it as a conversation between Tonto
and the Lone Ranger?". And that was when this book was really born.

After this the book seemed to take on a life all of its own and we both found
loads of energy for it. The characters of Tonto and the Lone Ranger seemed to
actually take over the book. They became real characters to us. Now we even
walk about wearing the clothes! I don't know what David's wife, Helen, thinks
about him going to bed in deerskins and a hunting knife, but Francesca has
been complaining loudly about me wearing my Texan hat and taking my six-
shooters to bed with me each night!

More seriously, though, we also wanted something that would express the
robustness of our relationship – a relationship that survived on humour and a
respect for the differences between us, just as the Lone Ranger and Tonto survived through a mutual respect of their different talents and of their different
cultures.

Ultimately, both David and I like to see ourselves as travelling the 'Wild West'
of bodywork and simply 'telling it how it is' - for us. Our aim is to help make
the land of Chair Massage a better place for everyone ...

That is our simple wish for this book.

We hope you enjoy reading it as much as we enjoyed writing it. We now place
you in the capable hands of the Lone Ranger and Tonto to lead you through the
land of Chair Massage ...enjoy!

Gerry Pyves, David Woodhouse

About horses, the Wild West, an Indian called Tonto and a Texas Ranger

———◆———

WE THOUGHT IT WOULD BE A GOOD IDEA to start with a brief description of these famous characters. So this is for those of you who were too young to be blessed with a childhood immersed in these archetypal and wondrously innocent role models ...

Created in 1933, the Lone Ranger and his Indian companion Tonto rode through the West bringing law and order during the Golden Age of radio and television (the TV show started in 1949).

The masked rider hid his identity because he was the lone survivor of a group of Texas Rangers ambushed by the Cavendish Gang. Tonto, a Potawatamie Indian, nursed him back to health and joined him in his crusade to bring law and order to the Wild West.

The American television show, starring Clayton Moore as the Lone Ranger and Jay Silverheels as Tonto, was one of ABC channel's biggest hits in the early 1950s.

Fans immortalised the show's most famous elements: the opening theme from "The William Tell Overture"; the Lone Ranger's wondrous horse, Silver, described by the show's announcer as "a fiery horse with the speed of light and thundering hooves"; Tonto's name for the Ranger, "Kemo-Sabe", meaning "trusted companion" (interestingly, the Lone Ranger first referred to Tonto in the radio series as Kemo-Sabe); the silver bullets; the Ranger's vow of refusing to shoot to kill and never removing his mask (unless in disguise).

Possibly the most enduring single icon of this show was the closing shot of the Lone Ranger shouting "Hi-Yo Silver!", whilst Silver pawed the air with his forelegs, both silhouetted against the setting sun ...

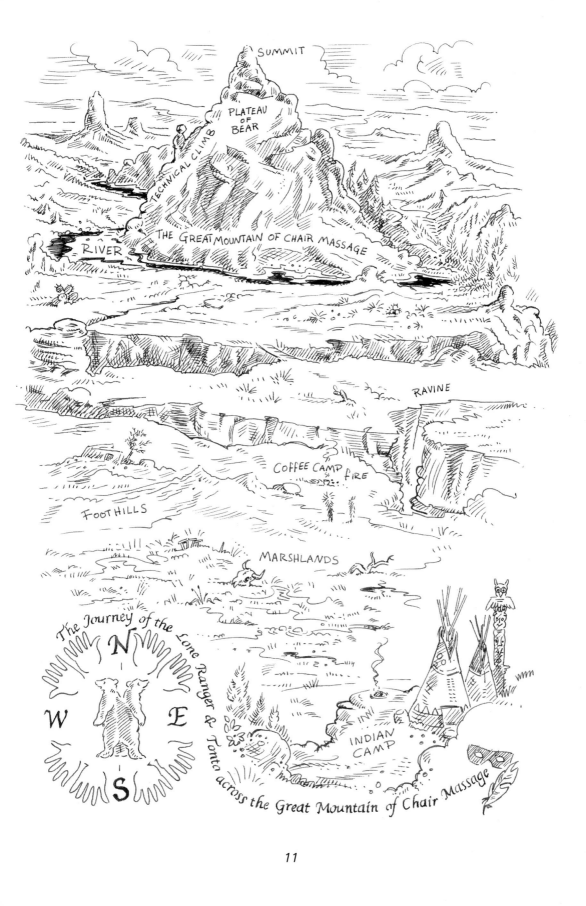

SUMMIT

PLATEAU OF BEAR

TECHNICAL CLIMB

THE GREAT MOUNTAIN OF CHAIR MASSAGE

RIVER

RAVINE

COFFEE CAMP FIRE

FOOTHILLS

MARSHLANDS

The Journey of the Lone Ranger & Tonto across the Great Mountain of Chair Massage

N

W E

S

INDIAN CAMP

1. LET'S JOURNEY ...

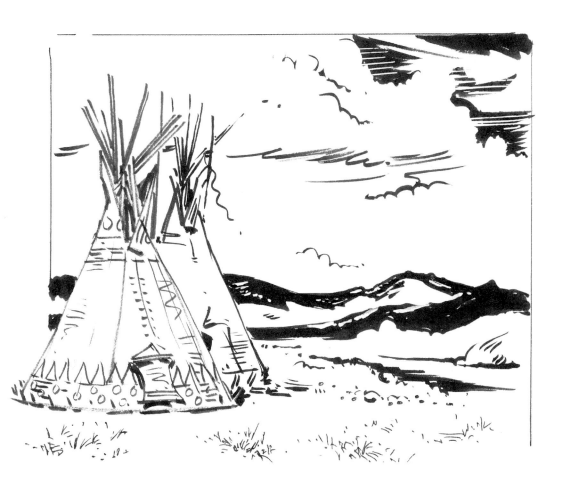

Packing our Bags

Kemo-Sabe?

Yes, Tonto?

Why are we writing to each other in this fashion with these names?

Well, Tonto ... you know how one of the ways I communicate what I do is through performances?

Oh yes, Kemo-Sabe! Your dances have set the massage world on fire!

Well, some people think I do it because I am a show-off ...

This is true, Kemo-Sabe

Thank you for that, Tonto

You are most welcome, Kemo-Sabe

Actually, the main reason for putting performances together was because, after 20 years of giving and watching demonstrations of bodywork,

I got bored ...

and I wanted to communicate my ideas and my approach in a way that was really interesting, inspiring and lots of fun for our practitioners. So I turned demonstration into theatre and found ways of massaging the audience's bodies while performing a massage with my co-performer on stage ... the whole thing was focused on reaching out and touching the people watching

Yes, and I was hypnotised and felt changed by what I saw, Kemo-Sabe!

I wanted actually to touch those practitioners who got involved in the performances, mentally, emotionally

And spiritually?

Yes! Those who chose to step out of their own world-view and lose themselves in an experience that celebrated touch itself – they were the ones who came up afterwards with tears in their eyes, saying it was the most moving thing they had ever seen as practitioners ...

And by inventing ourselves as Tonto and the Lone Ranger, you think we can do something similar?

Yes, I hope so. I hope that we can 'lighten up' a little with this approach, relax, enjoy and even have a little laughter together ...

Why is this so important, Kemo-Sabe? Won't people wonder why we have not presented our ideas in a serious academic format?

Well, Tonto, what I have learned from decades of training is that learning happens best when people are enjoying themselves. And massage doesn't have to be seen as so precious and fragile that we have to stay serious about the subject all the time

Well, bodywork is a serious business, Kemo-Sabe, and not something to be undertaken lightly ...

I know, Tonto, I know. In my work as a psychotherapist and as a bodyworker I have visited many dark places – suffering places that only the extreme depravity of the human psyche could have created – places that are so dark I would wonder if light were ever possible, or whether God ever existed …

Yes, Kemo-Sabe, I also have felt these places inside people's bodies – places where my clients have been hurt very badly

So, Tonto, when you have been in these places with your clients, and then, when you both come out of these dark places, and healing has transformed the darkness into pure light, what do you want to do, Tonto?

Why, Kemo-Sabe, when my client and I walk out of the dark cave into the fresh air and light, and once again hear the sounds of birds singing – we just want to cry with laughter and to dance and skip for joy!

So I want to write this book in a way that reflects the joy of healing touch

I like this idea very much, Kemo-Sabe!

Yes, Tonto, joy bubbles out of the painful places, after the wounds have been tended and dressed …

Then comes the laughter, Kemo-Sabe!

Yes, Tonto,

wild uncontrollable laughter

Yes, Kemo-Sabe, we laugh like children laugh

And this is true healing … because in the face of death and destruction and pain

We find the wellsprings of joy bubbling up!

Yes, and I wanted us to write a book that reflected some of this – some of our own journeys, as well as a technical book that covered some very new ideas. so that practitioners can not only get the information they need, but can enjoy the process

This is a lot for just one book, Kemo-Sabe!

Yes, it is. And it's also that I believe all bodywork is really about dialogue and I wanted to replicate a massage in the way we write this.

Don't you think massage is a dialogue between therapist and client, Tonto?

If you say so, Kemo-Sabe, but I prefer to work in silence whenever I can

Not that kind of dialogue, Tonto! I mean the kind of dialogue that means I lean into my client's tissues and they respond with a "Yes" or a "No" or a "Maybe?"

Perhaps the word "dance" does it better than dialogue.

Ah Yes, Kemo-Sabe, now I am with you. This dance you are talking about is what I call the "everlasting mating dance of the Mountain Eagle in the evening light"

Well, I would probably have to pass on the mating bit, Tonto, because we are dealing with professional practitioners who are ethical about their work, but "yes" to the poetry of your image

So how does this relate to our book, Kemo-Sabe?

Well, I thought it would be much more interesting for our whole book to be a dialogue between the two of us, so that people laugh and cry and travel with us and we let the conversation emerge and grow organically ...

Do you mean so that we can spar and lock horns like two crazy old rutting buffaloes in the mating season, Kemo-Sabe?

Look, Tonto, you are going to have to watch all this mating language – this is a book for some of the best and most serious practitioners in the world!

Oh ...

🌿 🌿 🌿

Kemo-Sabe?

Yes, Tonto?

Do they not mate also, these "best" and "serious" practitioners?

That's not the point, Tonto, Unless we keep it professional they will think we are not serious

But you are one of the most committed bodyworkers I know, Kemo-Sabe!

And so are you, Tonto, so let's not put people off, okay ?

Understood, Kemo-Sabe. I will be as circumspect as the She Wolf in heat, as cautious as the Mounting Rhino, as safe as the Wild Mountain Bear as he reveals himself to his mate and starts to ...

Tonto!

Sorry, Kemo-Sabe

So, Tonto, who shall we write this book for – who will travel with us?

Every bodyworker who wants to get out there and give touch to the world – who else

So shall we make it an erudite volume, this? Shall we dazzle them with all of our clever bodywork techniques and stun them with our expertise and references?

No, Kemo-Sabe, this is not necessary

So we can keep it playful and simple?

🌿 🌿 🌿

Tonto?

I am thinking, Kemo-Sabe ...

I think we can do whatever we want, Kemo-Sabe!

And, Kemo-Sabe, I know that I would very much like to read this book that you describe - it sounds full of nice things to keep me going along the difficult journey of reading it ...

So it is agreed then. We will write a bodywork book that is

fun!

Yes, Kemo-Sabe, all serious practitioners know how essential it is to laugh and cry in this land of bodywork

And, let us also honour them by ...

Getting right down to the really important "nitty gritty" of what they need to know?

Agreed!

Agreed!

So we want a book that is full of the same variety as exists in a bodywork session, where there can be stillness and seriousness and sometimes a need to giggle and laugh! Because Tonto, bodywork without laughter is like communion without wine ...

What do you think?

Perhaps it is the right time for a bodywork book that breaks the mould, just as your revolutionary NO HANDS approach has broken the mould of bodywork forever ...

You don't think we will upset anyone?

Kemo-Sabe, I think that all the bodyworkers who want to learn and laugh and dance will have plenty of fun with this book ...

Right then, let's do it!

Let us ride the Wild Panther into the darkness of the night, Kemo-Sabe!

No rutting, then Tonto?

Most definitely no rutting, Kemo-Sabe

Just one more thing, Tonto – is there anyone who this book is *not* for?

I think it is not for people who have no training in the basic tenets of traditional massage

I agree, Tonto. But why is this so important to you?

Because touch is so important, Kemo-Sabe!

If people have not learnt where the art of massage came from and how it developed and how it works with oil on skin and the power of traditional massage and all the many dangers and contraindications to touch, how can they ever be proper ambassadors of touch and apply these principles properly to clothed bodywork on chairs?

I think you're spot on my beautiful dear old hunting scout!

Can we put that into a box then, Kemo-Sabe?

The bit about you being a beautiful dear old hunting scout?

No, Kemo-Sabe - the bit about people needing to be trained in massage!

Yes! I think that is a great idea, Tonto

> If people have not learnt where the art of massage came from and how it developed and how it works with oil on skin and the power of traditional massage and all the many dangers and contraindications to touch, how can they ever be proper ambassadors of touch and apply these principles properly to clothed bodywork on chairs?

Kemo-Sabe, I am thinking that the evolution of all therapies must always begin with a solid grounding in the classic and it is then, and only then, that the practitioner can experiment – and take the past and develop it into the present and then the future ... and the future is most definitely Chair Massage.

Yes, Tonto, the future of bodywork has Chair Massage written all over it – which is why it is so important that training establishments like yours uphold the ancient traditions of massage as well as training people in the new traditions of Chair Massage.

There was never any question that we would continue the traditions of massage – by only training qualified massage practitioners.

When I started teaching NO HANDS Massage I also had the same dilemma of working out what level of therapist I would teach this to: should I train beginners or should I train graduates?

Whatever could have been gained from establishing a completely new approach for members of the public to learn massage from and train beginners. What would have happened to all the centuries of profound learning in bodywork if I had pursued this course of action?

It would have been like historical vandalism, Kemo-Sabe

Just so - we only truly stand upon the shoulders of giants when we acknowledge the thousands of years of human endeavour that precede our efforts ...

All those masters and their years of dedicated healing – their personal pain and sacrifice to discover the next great bodywork truth ...

All the way back to the Egyptians, the ancient Chinese and even back to the cave-dwelling healers ...

All the way back to the Ancient Ones, Kemo-Sabe ...

Yes. So, like you, I decided to teach only practitioners who had been trained in those massage traditions that form such deep roots in our bodywork tree - out of respect for the dedication of so many powerful and gifted touch healers..

You speak many words of wisdom, Kemo-Sabe and remind me of the saying "even within the dung of a camel, may pearls of truth be found"

Ummm ... was that a compliment?

Most certainly, Kemo-Sabe

Thank you, Tonto!

You are always most welcome, Kemo-Sabe!

Do you agree that this is one of those important bits that we need to put in a box?

About the camel dung, Kemo-Sabe?

No Tonto – about the training people need in order to do Chair Massage!

Just joking ...

I know. And the box?

Most assuredly a box, Kemo-Sabe

This book is only for qualified massage practitioners. If you do not know and have not learnt the 5 core strokes of Swedish Massage and have not learnt the anatomy and physiology of the body and the location of the muscles and the contraindications to massage and all the benefits of touch and massage, then put this book down now. Go and get the training your bodywork deserves! And then read on ...

So shall we begin, Tonto? I am keen to get going!

Just one small thing, Kemo-Sabe ...

Yes, Tonto?

You have not yet packed your bag

Oh dear! What shall I take, Tonto?

Certificates of Massage Qualification, Kemo-Sabe?

And?

All your previous knowledge and experience of bodywork, Kemo-Sabe

Including the past clients who have taught us so much?

Yes. And all the students who have asked important questions, Kemo-Sabe

Anything else?

Have you packed the map, Kemo-Sabe?

Ah yes – the map.....

And do not forget to pack lots of fun, Kemo-Sabe, for this is the food and water that will keep us going on this journey

Gotcha! So can we begin now, my wise old scout?

We have already begun. Now, let us ride the Black Panther into the darkness of the night, Kemo-Sabe!

Yes, let us treat this book like a journey, Tonto

And our destination, Kemo-Sabe?

I think our destination is the summit of the Great Mountain of Chair Massage. So what route shall we take?

Well, Kemo-Sabe, our way lies north, though it may sometimes feel as if we are getting nowhere, because we have to travel through some pretty nasty places – even across marshland

Yes, and won't there be some foothills to travel before we reach the summit?

Most assuredly, Kemo-Sabe! ... and there will be much difficult terrain, including ravines and difficult rivers, to cross

Okay Tonto, are we ready, now?

Most assuredly, Kemo-Sabe!

Then let us begin!

🌿 🌿 🌿

Oh, one more thing ...

Yes, Kemo-Sabe?

Thank you for travelling with me, Tonto

I wouldn't want to be anywhere else but here, Kemo-Sabe

The feeling's mutual, Tonto,

the feeling's mutual

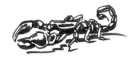

2. Into the
MARSHLAND
OF INJURY

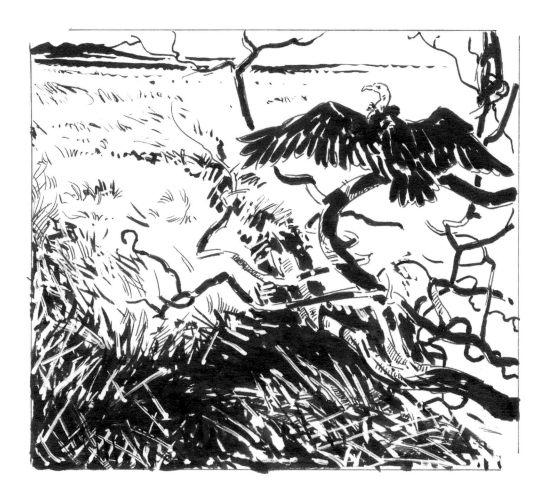

Kemo-Sabe?

    Yes, Tonto?

We have to start with an unpleasant bit of the journey first

    Why is that, Tonto?

So we can get directly into the mountains and move onto the more creative stuff, like the wonderful dance of Chair Massage...

    Tonto, can't we just avoid this. It would be much more comfortable going around the rocks. Look, there are some over there!

That is not the way. This injury thing is important, Kemo-Sabe

    I don't really have to go through it all again, do I? Can't I just let everyone read my other work? My first book, my articles? In fact, Tonto, you've even got some of this stuff in your saddlebag...

Kemo-Sabe ... it is a story that needs to be told over and over again – I will do it with you, for you are not the only one to find this subject unpleasant. Together we will get through this boggy land

    Thank you Tonto ... But do I really have to go through it all – it is very *heavy* stuff?

No, Kemo-Sabe let us not do this heavily – I will teach you how to walk lightly. Together, we will walk lightly through the marshes ...

    Mmmm ... walking lightly

                                      through this muck?

Like this, Kemo-Sabe ...

    Ugh! Do we really have to?

Yes, Kemo-Sabe

    Okay, after all, you're the scout, Tonto

Most assuredly, Kemo-Sabe

                                         🔥 🔥 🔥

Kemo-Sabe?

    Yes, Tonto?

I am right next to you – always

    Thank you, Tonto

You are most welcome, Kemo-Sabe

    So let's have a look at it as simply as we can, then Tonto ...

That is a good start, Kemo-Sabe

    We should really start with Newton's third law of motion

Which is?

"For every action there is an equal and opposite reaction"

What does this mean to practitioners of massage?

Well, Tonto, whenever we push or lean into the client's tissues, unless the client is pushed off the massage chair or table onto the floor, then it means that

the client's body resists and pushes our own weight back through our wrists

This means there are two forces meeting in our bodies – our own and the resistance of the client ...

This does not sound good, Kemo-Sabe

No! Especially when we do it over and over again ...

Aarghhh! Conventional bodywork techniques ... I call it trying to 'square the circle' – it is an impossibility!

Remember to walk lightly with me, Kemo-Sabe

Okay, okay, this is what I get all het up about.... Let me try again – lightly

Yes, lightly, Kemo-Sabe

mmmmmmmmmmm ...

You see, whenever we lean we create strain

and whenever we lean repeatedly, we create repetitive strain

Let us put this into a box, Kemo-Sabe:

> Simple movements that are normal, when
> repeated an abnormal number of times
> = repetitive strain injury.

It's all fundamentally due to a breakdown in the elasticity of the tissues in our body*.

---

* See *The Seven Stages of Injury*: Appendix p.138

Kemo-Sabe, what you say fits with my experiences. Our tutors had noticed for some time that hyper-extension of the wrist was beginning to cause problems already with some of our students and graduates. So we were already looking at injury-prevention techniques.

You were listening to your students and your graduates, Tonto – full marks!

Thank you. Our observations had been that some of the moves that had been handed down for centuries could be damaging to the practitioner ... and an injured practitioner is no good to his or her clients - just like when your own personal experience of injury threatened your career, Kemo-Sabe

Yes, Tonto – and do you recall my horror at looking at your thumb?

Yes, Kemo-Sabe - and your perverse delight in wanting to photograph it! I eventually succumbed to your request and it is reproduced in your manuals for all posterity to see. Okay, I admit that I was one of those who responded to your important study by saying that I had been experiencing problems with my hands and my wrists

It's nothing to be ashamed of, Tonto – having injured yourself by helping others. But there is so much to say about all this injury stuff that I feel as if I am sinking. Help!

Grab my arm! You see, Kemo-Sabe, you do not have to cover everything on your own – here give me some of that heavy information on injury, and I will put it into my saddlebag

You will carry my information on injury?

Yes, Kemo-Sabe. The ones who are unsure about this or want to find out more can turn to my saddlebag at the back of this book to follow it up later

Ah, that's much better. Look, I'm not sinking at all – neither are you!

I have had many years to learn how to walk lightly across these marshlands, Kemo-Sabe. There is just one more thing, though ...

Yes, Tonto?

We bodyworkers are sensitive souls and trained to be in tune with our bodies – won't we feel it hurting if it is injuring us so badly?

If only we could! Look at the injury diagram again and you will see that pain is experienced only at stage five of a seven-stage process. Go on, go back and have another look!

Walk lightly, walk lightly ... So this means that the first four stages of injury have already happened by the time we feel anything that can worry us?

Yes, Tonto. That is why I want to alert practitioners *before* they get injured

So Kemo-Sabe, what can we do to prevent this injury?

We can abandon the hands for all work that requires pressure. You see, Tonto, even if you leave a 48-hour gap between sessions, so that your tissues have time to recover properly, then ... the next time you massage, you injure yourself all over again - creating a further loss of elasticity and micro-tears.

And so it continues again and again. Look at what happens when we reach stage three on the diagram – and still we keep going!

Could this be why so many practitioners that I meet are run down, tired and exhausted, Kemo-Sabe?

Absolutely, because their bodies are constantly having to repair micro-injuries. It took me twenty years to work that one out, Tonto

The immune system of even the strongest person in the world would eventually buckle under that kind of pressure!

Just so, Tonto

If this is such a problem, why have we only heard about it recently through your work?

Well, it took many hundreds of years of nursing before they started to concern themselves about nurses' health, Tonto. And many, many typists were injured before they realised the full implications of repetitive movements creating long-term injury....

But a typist isn't applying anything like the pressure a massage practitioner is using all the time.

Yes, Tonto, we need to understand that what we are really talking about is the equivalent of a typist who is typing whilst doing a handstand!

So this is why you have been telling the massage world all about this, Kemo-Sabe?

Yes, Tonto. The point is this, you've got to ask the right questions. Instead of blaming myself for my injury I had to analyse why it had happened...and find solutions – and quickly!

Remember, I had a mortgage to pay ...

And while I was doing that, finding practical clinical solutions over here in the UK, there was also someone else - a woman called Lauriann Greene in the States. She was writing a book about how she was badly injured during her training and how she started running workshops in the States on hand protection with a whole load of exercises to prevent injury.....

This was done by a student, Kemo-Sabe?

Yes! For this she deserves great credit.

Like you, she refused to blame herself for her injuries, even as a student – do you think we should read this book, Kemo-Sabe?

Most definitely. And in it she coined a wonderful phrase "the massage athlete" which I love.

And what is this "massage athlete" that Lauriann Greene speaks of?

It means that unless we really treat ourselves in the same way as a professional athlete ...

You mean diet, exercise, stretching, training ...?

Exactly. Unless we do this we will not last the course

What sort of exercises would you recommend for injured hands, Kemo-Sabe?

None! I would recommend that therapists rest and stop massaging immediately they start to experience aches and pains, so that they can heal properly

No massage at all?

Well, none that involves the hand, Tonto. You see, with the approach of NO HANDS Massage I find that practitioners can actually speed up the healing process by working. But we digress

You see, Lauriann was brilliant .Her own personal massage boat crumpled against the iceberg of injury and she shouted,

"Iceberg!"

and quite wisely jumped ship and saved herself – and grabbed as many other practitioners out of the water as she could ... You see, she never actually took up the profession

I heard she was last seen driving around France tasting wines, Kemo-Sabe!

Not a bad life, Tonto, not a bad life at all. As for me, like a foolish captain with his ship and almost four years into full-time practice, I chose to go down with my boat!

This is a strange tradition for a Potawatamie Indian to understand, Kemo-Sabe, this sinking with your boat business. So how far did you sink?

A long way into injury, Tonto! And, as a result, I was able to examine the whole massive great injury iceberg as I sank deeper

and deeper

And this is how you learned about the seven stages of injury?

Yes, and the 200-year-old obsession that our industry has had with the hand ...

and I found out the likely demographic extent of this problem in our profession

Tell me more, about this, Kemo-Sabe

Well, Tonto, we asked a random group of practitioners whether they had been injured and of those that replied ...

78 per cent reported hand injury

Did you say 78 per cent, Kemo-Sabe?

Yep

So this injury statistic means that there have been a lot of wasted careers, Kemo-Sabe!

Yes, and the ones who are the very best – the ones who are becoming truly dynamic in their bodywork – these are the ones who will be most damaged

How so, Kemo-Sabe?

Because as they grow in confidence, practitioners begin to trust their own bodyweight more and use this to lean into the client's tissues.

Thereby putting more force through their wrists and fingers, Kemo-Sabe?

Yes. So our industry's obsession with the hand has meant that our most successful practitioners could become ... the most successfully injured!

So that is the whole iceberg, Kemo-Sabe?

Well, not quite Tonto. You see, we need to look at the history of massage. Did you know that within ten years of Swedish Massage arriving in America, in the 1850's, we see the invention of the first massage machines for the stated reason that practitioners were already reporting injury!

I did not know this, Kemo-Sabe

In your saddlebag, Tonto, you now have an article by me that explains how we are using Per Henrik Ling's Techniques in a way that he never intended......

Massage has changed then, Kemo-Sabe?

Yes. Massage has actually responded to the changes in society in a way no other therapy has done. It is attending to the massive stresses that our society is placing on people. We do this

with loooooooooooooooooooong

r   e   l   a   x   i   n   g

sessions

The massage practitioner of today is repeating movements many, *many times more* than they were ever designed fo ...

This is the rest of the iceberg, Kemo-Sabe?

Yes, this is what you really see if you get below the surface of our injury iceberg and reveal the true extent of the problem ...

You see, most massage is a very flexible and open profession – and sensitive practitioners adapt their treatments to their clients in a way that is simply not possible in more rigid healing systems ... responding to the massive social and technological changes within our society ...

And we may have seen more change to our daily lives in the last fifty years than in the previous 500.

Exactly, and the twentieth century also saw the biggest explosion of touch therapies the world has ever seen – a veritable therapeutic renaissance led entirely by bodyworkers. It is no accident that the two trends happened at the same time – massive social change and a renaissance of touch therapy

This makes right now the most exciting time in the history of the world to be a bodyworker!

So this is about a lot more than just injury prevention, isn't it, Kemo-Sabe?

Yup

And look, Kemo-Sabe, we have passed through the marshes and bogs and arrived at firm ground

By walking lightly, Tonto!

Yes, Kemo-Sabe, by walking lightly!

Well, I think I got a bit heavy in a few places, Tonto, and I would have sunk a few times if you hadn't held me up.

You did well, Kemo-Sabe; it was very boggy marshland we were travelling over

Yes, it is easy to get stuck in the bog ...Thank you for your help in guiding me through, Tonto – you are the best tracker in the world!

You are most kind, Kemo-Sabe

Tonto, can we climb those foothills over there?

Yes, Kemo-Sabe, if you are ready

Is it firm underfoot?

Yes, Kemo-Sabe

Good – I need to get my feet onto some of the really good stuff

So we can learn to dance like the Dancing Bear, Kemo-Sabe?

Yes. Tonto, this is what we need to do

Otherwise the Great Bear Spirit will not let us onto his sacred mountain

Nor should he, Tonto, nor should he ... So really, Tonto, this journeying is just preparation ...

An initiation, even

Yes, into the way of the dancing bear

That is correct, Kemo-Sabe, so let us keep going - we have a long way to go

Whatever you say, Tonto.

We travel through these foothills over here

So it is time to turn a few pages in the history of Chair Massage

That sounds exciting, Kemo-Sabe

Well, you are going to have to help guide me through this because we are covering a lot of ground in the next chapter, Tonto...

I am always by your side, Kemo-Sabe, and we can rest often ...

Tonto?

Yes, Kemo-Sabe?

I am glad we are out of the marshland!

Me too, Kemo-Sabe

And Tonto?

Yes, Kemo-Sabe?

I do not think I would have made it without you, thank you

You are most welcome, Kemo-Sabe

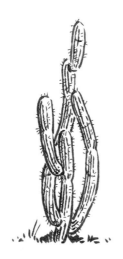

3. Into the Foothills of

CHAIR MASSAGE HISTORY

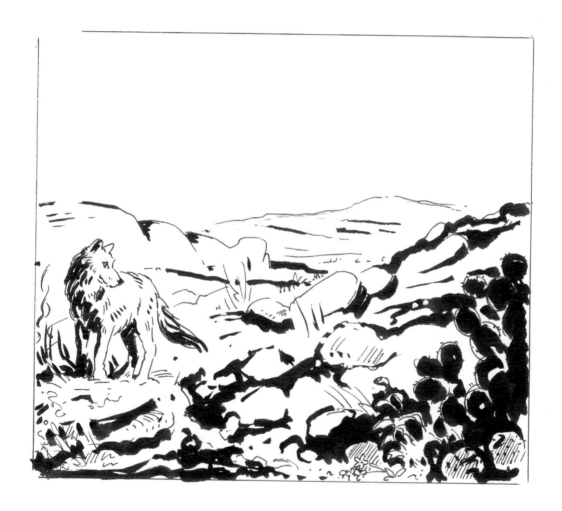

So, Tonto, let us get a firm footing by answering the important question about Chair Massage, namely where did it all appear from?

Well, Kemo-Sabe, the concept of seated massage was really given life in the USA through the inspirational work of David Palmer in 1982. He began training the graduates of his oriental acupressure school, the Anma Institute, in giving clothed 15- or 20-minute treatments of the back, neck and shoulders with the clients seated on chairs

Tonto, you do realise that almost all bodywork traditions have some experience and history of treating clients in a sitting position and of working through clothes?

Yes, Kemo-Sabe, centuries-old Japanese prints and even some ancient Egyptian engravings show people receiving massage while seated on low stools

And seated massage has been an integral part of Feldenkreis and Rolfing modalities (to name but two) for decades ...

In truth, Kemo-Sabe, individual practitioners have probably applied seated techniques to members of the public for as long as bodywork has been around

Even twenty years ago in my own training, Tonto, we did a whole module on clothed massage to clients in a sitting position so we could help people in everyday situations

Exactly, Kemo-Sabe. But what Palmer did was really to develop this idea in a way no-one else had ever done before. What was most revolutionary in what Palmer achieved was putting these all together (clothed and seated bodywork in public places) and in promoting this bodywork as a kind of brand to the public, making massage more palatable and accessible to thousands of people for the very first time. He coined the phrase "on-site massage" to differentiate it from the sort of massage that was going on in therapy rooms

So, just as MacDonald's made the American burger accessible to millions of people worldwide, Palmer made Chair Massage accessible to people all over the world?

Exactly, Kemo-Sabe – he even designed the first ever massage chair!

Yes Tonto, I now remember reading how one of the first companies to embrace this new 'bodywork in the workplace' concept and to buy Palmer's brand of bodywork was the highly innovative Apple Computer Company in Silicon Valley

Yes, at their peak, Palmer had seven practitioners offering 350 Chair Massages a week, all paid for by these trend-setting employers. The media became fascinated with this exciting development and Chair Massage was truly born. It is important to appreciate these historical and economical roots

Yes, it is very important to me to acknowledge the people who have really contributed to our profession's development ... standing on the shoulders of giants, and all that, eh, Tonto?

Yes, Kemo-Sabe. Chair Massage was, and still is, probably the biggest move our profession has ever taken on the offensive in the battle for public acceptability

of massage. For this alone, David Palmer deserves all the recognition he has got from the American Massage Association for services to the profession

You know, Tonto, I think that something like this has been needed by our profession for a long, long time: something that really gives the public a safe experience of the benefits of touch

Kemo-Sabe, can I quote Palmer himself on this whole issue of making massage acceptable?

Please do, Tonto

Well, Kemo-Sabe, Palmer once wrote:

> *"I have often noted that, if you wanted to make certain that professional massage would never become widely accepted in the Western culture, here is how it would be designed: force clients to go into a private room behind closed doors, take off all of their clothing, lay down on a table, and allow a stranger to rub oil all over the body ... There is only one other time when people get prone and naked behind closed doors with another person ..."*

Yes! How many practitioners have had to overcome this fear through building excellent rapport and trust so that clients can safely get naked on the plinth! I am often reminding practitioners of their extraordinary high skill level in making such behaviour safe for total strangers ...

Well, Kemo-Sabe, Chair Massage can now be seen in many public places – though it still has a long way to go in the UK. It really has made it safe for people to get touched and receive bodywork

Yes, there is actually something very safe about having bodywork in a public place – both for the client and the practitioner

Yes, Kemo-Sabe, working in a public place means that there are always witnesses, and the forward leaning position means the client is well protected......

Yes, almost a foetal position – and much less vulnerable than lying face up, naked on the plinth!

This is true, Kemo-Sabe

So what about the chair itself, Tonto? It always looks so good. Just seeing one of these chairs at an exhibition makes me think about all the benefits of massage. They look so sleek, so modern, so, dare I say it, kooool!

Well, Kemo-Sabe, by May 1986 the first production models of Palmer's design of the seated massage chair began. And there are now twenty manufacturers around the world who have produced in excess of 100,000 chairs - all

developments of Palmer's original design. Every year the design seems to get a little better and a little more comfortable – just like the evolution of the aeroplane...

So that's how this icon of the public face of massage became almost a brand in its own right, Tonto. The chair now signifies relief from tension and instant relaxation. I believe it is probably one of the most market-friendly inventions our profession will ever witness. Just to see a chair standing alone is to invite interest and enquiry.....

Yes, Kemo-Sabe, which is why it is such an important tool for practitioners to come to terms with and learn how to use properly – both for their own marketing and for the good name of our profession

So Tonto, we have public massage, we have clothed massage and we have a new chair designed specifically for bodywork. What else was innovative about Palmer's work?

Well, Kemo-Sabe, David Palmer also coined the phrase "entry-level massage". He used this to distinguish this simple level of bodywork (lasting only 15-20 minutes) from the more profound and deep bodywork that takes place in the privacy of the consulting room - and can last for over an hour

So, for all Chair Massage, the intention is simply relaxation and health enhancement?

Yes, Kemo-Sabe. The purpose of Chair Massage is to bring touch out into the public arena and thereby expose touch as a healthy thing. David Palmer talks of his vision of achieving a situation where

"Touch is recognised as essential to the development and maintenance of healthy human beings ..."

This "entry-level massage" aims to provide a short space in which clients can relax and recharge in the middle of their work, conference or shopping excursion. It is designed to relax and loosen muscles, and to provide a rebalance or even a recharge of energy through working the meridians

And that is what the practitioner aims to achieve?

Yes, Kemo-Sabe, because anything too deep could leave the client disorientated or even in a state of emotional distress or confusion

Yes – the power of touch is profound. It's almost as if we have to protect those clients whom we see in the public arena from the whole power of touch, isn't it?

Yes, Kemo-Sabe – hence the phrase "entry-level massage"

In my first ever article on Chair Massage, I questioned the appropriateness of giving bodywork to people in public environments or in the dog-eat-dog atmosphere of the corporate workplace

Your concerns were for the well-being of the clients receiving touch in such environments?

Yes, Tonto. And I explained that it was no accident that healers and physicians have required their clients to come to their own offices or clinics for thousands of years. They did this to be in total control of the environment

Yes, Kemo-Sabe, and many Chair Massage practitioners seek to retain this control, often finding private rooms to work in even when in office or corporate environments

So when I wrote my article in 1986 at the very birth of Chair Massage, I was concerned about two things. Firstly, I did not understand why it was called massage when it was seated clothed acupressure, and secondly, I was concerned about the environments in which it took place

This was before you knew about "entry-level massage"?

Yes, and after writing that article, I remember having a very robust argument with one of my former students of massage, Mike Zimmerman, who went over to San Francisco to train with David Palmer and now teaches Chair Massage in the UK. It was he who introduced me to this concept of "entry-level massage"

And since then?

Well, I have come to appreciate the enormous value of providing "entry level massage" to the community. At the time I was in fact providing a similar approach to massage myself. I was running a community massage project in Manchester in which members of the public were being taught to give a basic and introductory level of massage touch to each other in supervised environments

So, like Palmer you also were trying to get touch out there into the community?

Like so many other bodyworkers who have had the privilege of personally experiencing the amazing power of touch to heal and soothe our ragged lives...We just want to reach out to the public and say:

> *"For God's sake, stop taking those pills and eating that junk and putting that stuff into your body – just try this and let the most powerful medicine on the planet, touch, heal your life ... "*

Yet there is so much power in touch, and our society has become so starved of it, that there is a very real ignorance of the impact that even the simplest of touch can produce – which is why I believe that public bodyworkers need to be absolutely clear about the scope and boundary of their work

What is your point, Kemo-Sabe?

Well, from my own experiences, I know that sometimes the most incredible transformations can take place for people even when the practitioner is simply focusing on relaxation

Yes, Kemo-Sabe, life-changing moments can occur for people through the power of simple touch

Anyone who has worked as a bodyworker knows this, and we can do nothing to stop this powerful effect of touch – even if we wanted to

I understand, Kemo-Sabe. I am not sure a bodyworker has the right to deny people this powerful healing

Nor am I, Tonto. It is my belief that the client is in charge of what happens to them internally and what use they put the massage to. The practitioner is only responsible for what he or she actually does and that comes down to having a clear intention ...

An intention simply to relax and provide the benefits we have already discussed?

Yes, Tonto. The stronger the conscious and stated intention of the practitioner, the more likely the client is simply to take what is being offered – "entry-level massage". Yet this will never prevent the client from taking a whole lot more, if they need it – whatever the practitioner does

Yes, Kemo-Sabe, life is not always a conscious thing. I believe that there is a body wisdom within the client that sometimes says, "Yes, I need this touch to bring me back into harmony". This has nothing to do with either the conscious intention of the practitioner or the client

It is true that we are dealing with so much more than simply the conscious intention when it comes to touch. When we touch another human being we touch both their conscious and their unconscious being

This is why bodywork sometimes resembles a dream, Kemo-Sabe?

Yes, Tonto, and like a dream, we cannot always control the outcomes ... Tonto! why are you lying on the ground?

Hide behind this rock, Kemo-Sabe, quickly! Someone is coming ...

How many people are there, Tonto?

Just one Kemo-Sabe, carrying a 40lb-back-pack, sweating profusely and breathless – also wearing a big brown hat and carrying two six-shooters in cross-slung holsters!

That is incredible, Tonto! How do you tell all this just from simply listening to the ground?

I didn't, Kemo-Sabe, I just saw him walking up the hill!

Tonto!

Sorry, Kemo-Sabe, I could not resist it

Ah, I know this person, Tonto. He is one of my Chair Massage students, called Ruaring Massage Brave. Greetings!

Hello, Masked Ranger, we meet again - and greetings, Tonto! It is great to meet you at last; I have heard so much about your good work

How!

Where are you headed?

I am travelling to the mountains in the north to meet up with my pardner Judy

I did not realise you were in these parts. Have you been here long?

You of all people should know that – after all it was you who showed me how to get here and what a great land it is. I guess it's about a year

Listen, Ruaring Massage Brave, have a drink of water and rest a few minutes. Maybe you can help Tonto and me with something we are debating

Well, I am rather thirsty ... Ah, that's better. Thank you, Tonto

Kemo-Sabe and I are talking about "entry-level massage"

And we are discussing the problem of keeping the client as safe as possible ...

Whilst at the same time giving them all the powerful benefits of touch

You know, I have really struggled with this part of Chair Massage. In all my individual therapeutic massage sessions at my clinic ...

Which last about an hour?

Yes, somewhere between 40 minutes and an hour ... Well, in all these sessions, I aim to make my work as powerful and as potent as possible – so that my clients can really get all the help that touch offers them

And with your Chair Massage?

Well, in the busy hospital environment where I work, I still do not like to hold myself back

So you do not actually practise" entry-level massage"?

I hope you will not be offended, Masked Ranger, but I remember you teaching this to me and at the time it sounded good. In practice, however, I found it was an idea that restricted my bodywork

So you abandoned it?

Yes

So how do you work instead?

I allow myself to go very deeply just for a couple of minutes – and longer only if I feel the client needs and responds positively to this

And this is safe for the client? Don't your clients then go into a deep space that is hard for them to come out of?

Well, very rarely. Remember that I explain to them the simple scope of the bodywork right at the beginning of each session, so most of them take the session at that level

You are programming them in advance to accept and expect "entry-level massage"?

Yes, Tonto

So what if they do visit a deep and powerfully healing place?

Then this is because they needed to go there!

But what of the client's ability to come back into the important world of, say, accident and emergency care?

Well, this is fascinating to both myself and Judy, because all our people walk through the rooms of the Chief Executive of the hospital on their way into and out of our sessions

Wow! Instant assessment or what! This is the harsh reality of this corporate land – results are sometimes very public!

Most assuredly, Kemo-Sabe, if this work does not produce miracles immediately, it does not survive. The big chiefs always want to see what is going on

That's right, Tonto. For myself and Judy, we realised very early on that our very survival in this land depends on what people are seeing our touch actually achieve – which is why I do not like the idea of giving anything less than 100 per cent to our sessions, something we can do with your zero-strain approach, Masked Ranger

And the clients that walked out of your sessions through the Big Chief's rooms?

Well, whether they had visited a deep space or not, they looked great! Far from looking more tired, the depth and potency of the bodywork seemed to re-energise them. I would say that the deeper the experience – the greater the release of energy. And every day the waiting list of people wanting our Chair Massage grows because of this

Is this not the true power of touch, Kemo-Sabe?

Yes it is, Tonto. And you cannot stop people from taking what they need from touch – even if you wanted to! I remember doing 2-3 minutes of massage on people at an exhibition and telling them (sometimes having to shout close to their ears because of all the noise around us!), telling them that this was just a demonstration of the physical force that NO HANDS makes available to the practitioner

And what happened, Kemo-Sabe?

Well, the vast majority felt great and that was it. But one woman came back the next day and brought three of her friends to have these two-minute sessions and told me that during her touch session she had a really powerful experience and – for the first time ever, had really let go and said goodbye to her father – who had died three years ago!

All this in a busy exhibition hall, Kemo-Sabe!

Yes Tonto, and all I was doing was concentrating on providing safe, firm touch

But Kemo-Sabe, for three years she had been preparing herself to do this letting go?

Yes Tonto, and as practitioners we have no idea what unconscious agendas our clients may have

All of us who do Chair Massage have witnessed something of this power of touch, Kemo-Sabe, and it is good never to restrict the scope of our work.

More than that! We should not be afraid to give our clients really powerful touch. What Judy and I found was that far from restricting our work, we would just let it flow wherever it wanted to – and consequently we had loads more energy ourselves

Even when following our Kata, it is possible to work very deeply with people – sometimes the bodywork just takes over.

That's what we found, Tonto! I guess it's important to say also that we did not place any pressure on ourselves to do anything more than just a good solid piece of bodywork whilst those who needed more took more, whatever we did – there were sessions where I clearly gave more. Perhaps some of this was because they were more receptive to touch and I was willing to give more.

Whatever they took from the session, they all looked and felt great!

So your very best marketing is the power of your massage and the visible effects it is having on the clients?

Yes. Once we had done all the hard work of actually getting ourselves into the hospital in the first place, it was only the reputation of our bodywork that kept us there.

And you are sure that the clients were not tired or exhausted?

No, Masked Ranger; in fact they were even more energised!

This makes a lot of sense to me. You see this happen a lot in any massage. It's as if all the physical tension we use literally to "hold ourselves together" also exhausts us energetically. Once we let go and release this tension through simple touch, all that locked-up energy becomes available to us, so we can perform our daily tasks much better

Yes, Kemo-Sabe! In our work we have a way of describing this also: we say that exhaustion stems from a blockage of the body's Ki.

And because the practitioner releases this blockage, the client has more Ki or energy available?

Exactly, Kemo-Sabe. More specifically, the meridians are like rivers that run through the body.

Imagine a log jamming the river. This is like the blockage to the flow of Ki in our bodies. It is tiring for us to deal with these blockages.

So, when we touch the tsubo, it's as if we nudge the log out of the way and the flow of the river disperses the blockage

And the river flows freely, releasing all that blocked energy to complete our daily tasks?

That is right, Kemo-Sabe

That is a beautiful description of bodywork, Tonto

Thank you, Ruaring Massage Brave

And it explains why deep and relaxing Chair Massage bodywork leaves the client more energised at the end!

And why your clients walking though the Big Chief's rooms are so radiant and full of the joys of life, Ruaring Massage Brave

Yes, Tonto

Ruaring Massage Brave?

Yes, Tonto?

Could you tell us more about your work in this hospital? It sounds so exciting

I would love to Tonto, but Judy really does await me in the mountains due north of here and I have already delayed my journey too long, I really must leave you now – and your journey is still a long and hard one. That is a very hard mountain to climb, that great mountain of Chair Massage!

I am sad at your leaving

Me too, Tonto, but I am sure we will meet again. Actually, I have something here that will fit into your saddlebag. It is an account of our work in this hospital, so you can read it after I have gone. Perhaps it will help you on your journey

You are most generous. Thank you!

Well, Tonto, you of all people know that "what you give is what you get"

Most assuredly, Ruaring Massage Brave. Farewell!

Farewell, Tonto, farewell Masked Ranger

Farewell, and good luck to both you and Judy!

Ꭿ Ꭿ Ꭿ

I liked this Ruaring Massage Brave. Was he a good student, Kemo-Sabe?

One of the best, Tonto, one of the very best

Kemo-Sabe?

Yes, Tonto?

What if a client comes actually stating that they want a therapeutic treatment or session?

Well, I believe that a client who seeks something deeper at the outset is a different matter. If he or she wishes for more from the bodywork than simple health enhancement, or relaxation, then the practitioner must always ensure that this can actually be delivered and the client is in the right environment

I agree with this, Kemo-Sabe. Many Chair Massage practitioners actually give

deeper therapeutic treatments in corporate settings, but they are in private rooms ...

This is the difference between a public and private massage, Tonto. Public Chair Massage should always aim for health enhancement only.

In the privacy and security of the consultancy room, however, so much more can be agreed to beforehand. The main thing here is that the client has time and space to make the transition from the sometimes dream-like world of touch back into work.

Even in the workplace there are private offices, Kemo-Sabe, and it is possible to give longer and deeper treatments. When the session has gone very deep, a few minutes and a glass of water will often suffice

Well, maybe. But I am fundamentally uncomfortable about this sort of session taking place in the workplace from the outset. Chair Massage seems to be at its weakest when it tries to mimic therapeutic sessions in a practitioner's consultancy room. If clients have a powerful physical or emotional reaction to the massage, then they must be in an environment that is safe enough for them to come round slowly and not to suffer ridicule from their colleagues. It is a very delicate thing. For this reason, I believe that anyone seeking a therapeutic outcome of any depth should be referred to a longer individual session in the privacy of the clinic

So it is about intention?

Yes, I believe the intention for Chair Massage has to be for relaxation and general health enhancement – no matter how powerfully that is given by the practitioner

And this is where Chair Massage has several distinct advantages over conventional massage, does it not?

Yes, Tonto, it is time to really speak out loudly about these. So what is your favourite advantage of Chair Massage over table massage?

Well, Kemo-Sabe, I like very much that this work can be done anywhere and certainly falls within the category of prevention rather than cure

Yes, Tonto, much bodywork takes place after someone has already become stressed at work. Chair Massage can actually reduce stress in the very place it is happening – giving the tension less time to lock into the tissues and cause its damage

What about you, Kemo-Sabe, What do you like most about Chair Massage?

Well, after twenty years of persuading people to book sessions well in advance and then to take off their clothes and be covered in oil, I love the fact that they can just climb onto the chair and have a session – so simple!

Yes, Kemo-Sabe, it appeals to many people who would not otherwise contemplate a massage for themselves ...

And is therefore promoting touch to the world in a way that conventional and private bodywork never could

And because the session is so short and so accessible, Kemo-Sabe, people who may not yet prioritise their health enough to book an hour and travel to a therapist are often quite willing to have a short Chair Massage session

And because of its short duration, Chair Massage is also exceedingly popular

Yes, amazingly, it works in conditions where you would normally never expect massage to be able to work!

And, Tonto, let us not forget that it does actually deal with most of the obvious external manifestations of stress: you know, muscular tension, congested meridians, aching muscles, tightly held joints etc...

Yes, Kemo-Sabe, and who knows what internal benefits? And, in contrast to most stress management approaches in the work-place, it requires little action from the client – they just get to sit there and get de-stressed!

Yes, Chair Massage really does get touch out there and into the public domain in a way that looks professional and attractive

It helps rid the profession of the sleazy image that has haunted our profession for so long.

Amen to that, Tonto! It means that practitioners can really do something to help their profession by learning Chair Massage and getting out there into the public domain

Kemo-Sabe?

Yes, Tonto?

More people are coming!

What can you see?

Clouds of dust from two riders, Kemo-Sabe – over there

I can see them – looks like they are coming this way. Why is this part of the land so busy?

These foothills provide access to many different parts of this land, Kemo-Sabe

A sort of crossroads? So that explains it. Shall we hide?

No Kemo-Sabe, they look friendly and have no guns. Look, they are waving at us!

I know these two! It's Petrissage Pete and his hunting scout, Running Water. They were in one of my monthly practitioner support groups for many years – when I was first developing NO HANDS Massage. They were two of the pioneers who were trying out my approaches on their clients – with great results. It was because of their positive feedback and the reported feedback of their clients that I found the courage and the strength to carry on – even when people were saying, "NO HANDS Massage – are you mad?"

Some of us already know that you are truly demented, Kemo-Sabe

Thank you for that, Tonto

You are most welcome, Kemo-Sabe. Those pioneering days must have been

exciting, Kemo-Sabe

Pioneering *years*, Tonto, years. It took me over ten years finally to go public with the techniques and approaches that I had been showing to these groups.

Look, here they are now. Hail friends!

> *Whoa! Howdy Lone Ranger – what you doing so far north?*

Tonto here is taking me to the great mountain of Chair Massage in the North, to apply NO HANDS approaches to this area of massage. What about you two – what are you up to?

> *Running Water and I are going off to the West – Looking at Chair Massage in cancer-care environments*

Will you stop with us for a while? Tonto here brews a wicked black coffee

> *Who can resist such an offer? Come on, Running Water, it's time we took a break, anyway*

So tell me what you two are up to?

> *Well, Lone Ranger, as you know I have always been interested in finding research that can prove how wondrously therapeutic this bodywork is for people*

This work you do, this research, is so important

> *Well, thank you – we all have our part to play in this exciting enterprise*

Yes, we do. I even heard that you went to visit the great guru of massage research, Dr. Tiffany Field? She is doing such an important job in demonstrating and proving the benefits of touch to a very sceptical group – the medical establishment. That is a tough road to travel

> *Yes, Lone Ranger, Tiffany Field was an inspiration. But don't be too harsh on the medical establishment. They receive government funding and have to show scientific evidence for practically everything they decide to allocate funds for*

I suppose that cannot be easy for them. So what proof have you discovered?

> *Well, we now have some very strong evidence to prove many of the benefits that you have been talking about for years*

This is exciting! So tell us, have you found any evidence for the increased alertness and effectiveness that people who actually receive Chair Massage report after a session? We have just been discussing this

> *Absolutely! One recent study has actually shown Chair Massage reduces stress and enhances the electroencephalogram brain patterns for alertness in subjects. Another showed reduced anxiety levels, as well as improved alertness, that actually resulted in higher scores in computational tasks after treatment than in a control group*

So the combination of relaxation and alertness has been shown to be helpful for people?

> *Absolutely*

Any other findings? What about people just feeling more nurtured and supported?

> *Well, Running Water and I did our own study on this one and came up with excellent results that showed how people experienced positive effects from all this help and attention. It lifted their moods. Interestingly, this was also associated with the postural support that Chair Massage provides*

So your research showed a connection between physical support being experienced as emotional support as well?

> *I think some of our results could be interpreted that way, yes. This might explain another study in the States that showed over 85 per cent of participants experiencing both emotional and physical stress reductions. In the UK relatives of those in care also reported similar effects on mood. Another study showed that with enhanced well-being came greater emotional control. Yet another showed significant decreases in levels of anxiety*

This is fascinating – showing that touch can help people to be more in control of their emotions?

> *It looks that way, doesn't it?*

What about the physical benefits? You mention postural support.

> *Well, in addition to the more obvious and observable muscular benefits, we also have strong evidence for Chair Massage **lowering blood pressure**, decreasing the incidence of **sleep disturbance**, and actually **reducing pain**. There is also evidence for clear improvements in circulation*

This is fantastic! We should make sure that everyone is told about this. Every Chair Massage practitioner should be publicising this stuff. Will you stay and tell us more about all this?

> *Well, I would love to stay and talk more, but I am afraid that Running Water and I have to be going now - we are already behind schedule for some important projects. Thank you for that coffee Tonto, it was superb*

I am very sad that you cannot stay and spend more time with us, Petrissage Pete. I would love to hear more about all this research

> *Well now, it just so happened that Running Water and I did hear rumours that you were travelling in this part of the country. So we brought along a special document for you to take away with you – as a gift. Here it is, Tonto – put it in your saddlebag to read later. Catch!*

You are most generous, both of you!

> *Our pleasure – keep up the good work! Come on, Running Water, we have a long way to go. Farewell!*

Blessings on your journey. Farewell!

> Goodbye and good luck!

Kemo-Sabe?

Yes, Tonto

That was a good man

Yes, both Petrissage Pete and Running Water are doing truly important work. It takes real dedication to give so generously and see these research projects through to the bitter end. Talking of which – how are we doing?

We have come to the ravines and must move much more carefully now. Are you ready?

Yes, Tonto, I enjoyed the Foothills of Chair Massage history. Are these ravines dangerous?

Well, Kemo-Sabe, we must tread carefully

And stick together?

Always we must stick together, Kemo-Sabe

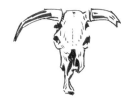

4. Into the Ravine of

BODYWORK LINGUISTICS

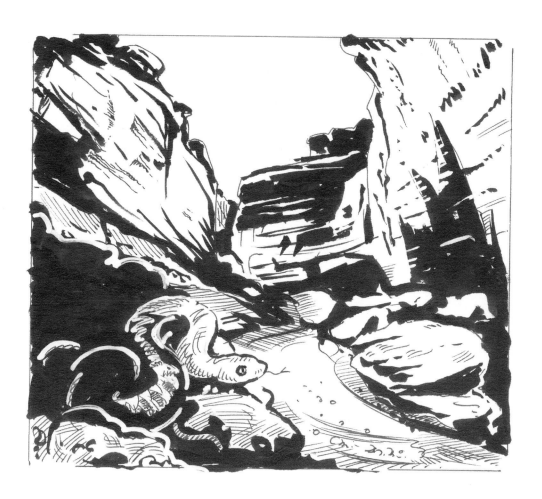

So, Tonto, would you agree that because of the training and expertise of the founder of seated massage, David Palmer, a great deal of Chair Massage training and literature has been focused on the use of acupressure techniques?

Yes, because that was what he was an expert in, Kemo-Sabe

Then we need to bring some new balance to the Chair Massage story and make a distinction between two very different traditions of bodywork

How do you mean, Kemo-Sabe?

Well, I believe that the profession's use of language has got a bit sloppy in describing what is going on in Chair Massage

Such as?

We need to make a distinction between what is, in effect,

meridian-based bodywork

and what could be more accurately described as

muscle-based bodywork

You see, Tonto, all good bodyworkers will be having a significant impact on both the *meridian flow* and the *muscle tone*, but it is important to the profession to understand the different *routes* by which we get there – in the same way as we need to know the difference between a train and a helicopter when travelling to a particular destination

But, Kemo-Sabe, I thought you always travelled by horse? Those wild angry iron horses and thes screaming fire bird machines are most distressing to the gentle skunk and the rutting musk rat ...

If you say so, Tonto, but could we stay focused on our bodywork discussion?

Sorry, Kemo-Sabe,

Well, Tonto, the point is this: different methods of transport result in different experiences, even though the destination arrived at may be the same.

Most assuredly, but do not speak so loudly of these infernal machines within the hearing of Silver, Kemo-Sabe. He is a jealous horse ...

All right ... So, no matter how similar the *end results* are, we need to be able to discuss the methods of getting there accurately

So, we need to have an in-depth understanding of the different approaches and intention and training of, say, muscle-based and meridian-based therapists?

Yes!

And Chair Massage is a good place at which to get clear about these two different approaches to bodywork?

Yes, Tonto, I think it is essential to our understanding of Chair Massage

Okay, then, Kemo-Sabe, can you tell me more about this difference between

muscle-based bodywork and meridian-based bodywork?

Well, simply put, the meridian-based bodyworker is trained to change the client's health through stimulating or altering the Ki picture of the client's energy. This is done through pressing along the meridians – often on specific *tsubo* or points. Some schools of thought do this by pressing into the meridian, and some by stretching the meridian and lowering the practitioner's HARA close to the client's meridians

And some with a combination of the two, Kemo-Sabe...

Yes, whereas the muscle-based bodyworker, is trained to alter the *tone* and *elasticity* of the muscles in order to impact on the structural balance and overall health and well-being (energy) of the client. This is done largely through *kneading* the muscles

Whichever discipline you were trained in, be it meridian-based (oriental acupressure work on meridians) or muscle–based (Western massage training on muscles), one of the most useful models that I and my students find for understanding what we are actually doing is in the next diagram.

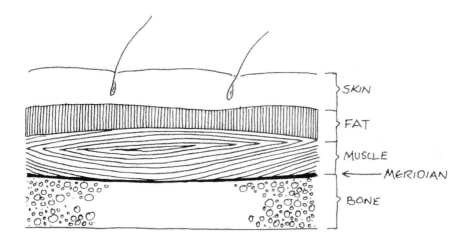

Now, Tonto, I don't know what you think, but most acupressure, shiatsu and acupuncture practitioners say one of the following three things in answer to the question: "Where exactly is the meridian?"

a) alongside the major nerves and blood vessels

b) inside the muscles

c) between the muscles and the bones

Well, Kemo-Sabe, when I am pressing into the tsubo I know that I have to press through skin and fat and muscle in order properly to contact the meridian, so this very much fits what I teach my students ...

Okay. Now the truth is that no-one really knows where the meridians are. If anything they travel through all the different tissues of the body. This diagram is obviously a gross over-simplification, but it is one that *works* for understanding different approaches to bodywork.

Because we all know that meridians can go deep into the central organs of the body and emerge close to the surface at other places in the body, particularly the limbs

Yes. Fascinatingly, we also find that both types of bodyworker (muscle-based or meridian-based) are achieving their results by working both deeply *and* superficially

Kemo-Sabe, it's as if acupressure and massage are approaching the same peak, but from two different sides of the mountain!

Which is why we will need to climb very high to get a proper view of this terrain. So let's put that in a box.

> It's as if acupressure and massage are approaching the same peak – but from two different sides of the mountain

So the muscle-based bodyworker addresses the tension primarily in the muscle layers. Now it is my experience that one thing that really shuts down the flow of Ki through the meridians is *muscle tension*.

We should imagine the tight muscles pressing the meridian against the bone and strangling it?

Yes, and sometimes strangling the meridian as it runs through it. Nor should we forget that muscle tension is one of the more obvious ways in which our mental and emotional state manifests itself in the body. If I am upset, then my stomach muscles harden first and then my *Hara* is congested and the flow of Ki throughout all my meridians is reduced …

Because the muscles constrict the actual meridians?

Yes. Our muscles have been shown to respond directly to the messages from our brains. Likewise, as the muscles relax through *massage*, so the constriction on the *Hara* and the meridians is released. This is why loosening the muscles has such a powerful impact on our minds

Not so much the mind-body link as the mind-muscle link?

Exactly. When we really get down to it, the mind-body link is largely expressed through our muscles contracting or releasing

Causing a constriction or release of Ki throughout the client's body!

Yes. And with meridian-focused bodywork, what is happening is that we find all sorts of clever ways to press through the tight muscle in order to contact and stimulate the meridian flow

Yes, Kemo-Sabe – the great skill in meridian-based bodywork is learning how to sneak through that tight muscle and contact the meridian

And as the meridians start to rebalance and the Ki starts to flow …

The muscles relax!

Yes, Tonto, muscle-based bodywork releases muscles *first* and the meridian flow changes as a *secondary* effect, whilst meridian-based bodywork releases meridian flow *first* and the muscles relax as a *secondary* effect

I think that should go in a box, Kemo-Sabe

Okay, here it is:

Muscle-based bodywork releases muscle first and the meridian flow changes as a secondary effect,

whilst

meridian-based bodywork releases meridian flow first and the muscles relax as a secondary effect

---

So this is why it is important to learn a little precision in our language?

Yes. Then, when we use these descriptions of bodywork, we know exactly what we are talking about

How does all this look when we examine what is actually happening to the client during a session, Kemo-Sabe? What differences does an onlooker actually see?

Okay, so if we take a problem like a very tight upper back, where the muscles are very hard and there is restricted movement …

Well, here the meridian-based bodyworker would seek to contact the meridians using point work and stretches …

What an observer would see is the practitioner gently pressing and leaning into the *tsubo* along the meridian – agreed?

Yes, and an observer would see the practitioner working all down the back and arms, not necessarily focusing on the tight muscles in the back

Now, by contrast, the muscle-based bodyworker would seek to restore softness to the muscle tissues themselves

And what the onlooker would see is more kneading and working of the large

muscle areas, rather than specific points?

> Yes

Kemo-Sabe, has this distinction between meridian-based and muscle-based bodywork ever been made before?

> Well, I haven't seen it in the literature, and it could pave the way for real clarity of description for practitioners and clients alike. I am not interested in making one sort of bodywork better than another. All I am trying to do is to use language accurately

Mmmm ... I like this linguistic distinction, Kemo-Sabe. You have just simplified so many different types of bodywork – perhaps all bodywork can be put into one of these two categories?

> Whoa there, Silver!

Kemo-Sabe, how could you?

> I'm sorry, Tonto. But I don't think we can lump together all bodywork ... this renaissance in new touch therapies - I am not sure that they could all be squeezed into just two categories, Tonto – for example, what about all the subtle energy work, and Reiki and cranio-sacral bodywork?

Yes, there are more colours to this profession than in the female dragonfly's bottom ...

> Talking of which, Tonto ...

We are out of the Ravine, Kemo-Sabe!

> With a new way to describe Chair Massage, Tonto?

Most definitely, Kemo-Sabe

> But what have we here?

It is a river, Kemo-Sabe

> And ... ?

We must cross it!

> I thought you might say that

⫸◦⫷

5.
CROSSING THE RIVER

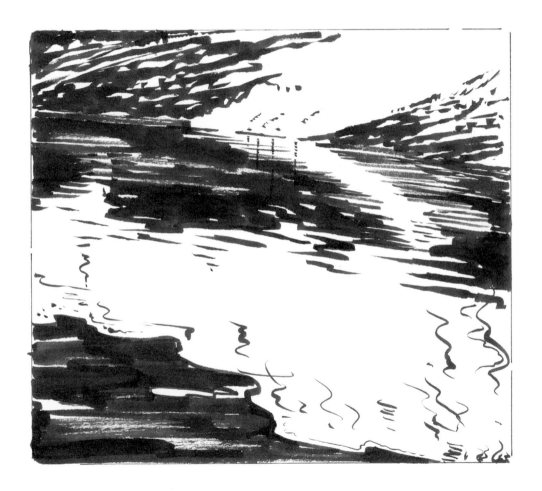

of Massage Evolution

So, Kemo-Sabe – we have established that conventional massage techniques are now creating all sorts of injury problems for practitioners

Yes, Tonto – that little secret is well and truly out the closet now!

And we have seen how Chair Massage first evolved, and some of the linguistic problems it has faced us with.

Yes, Tonto

But, Kemo-Sabe, tell me, what does all this mean for Chair Massage?

Okay, Tonto – you were trained in conventional massage before you learned Chair Massage, yes?

Do you mean that I trained in muscle-based bodywork before I learnt my meridian-based bodywork?

Exactly

Yes, Kemo-Sabe, this is true

Well, do you use your thumbs and fingers more or less in Chair Massage?

More, Kemo-Sabe

And do you lean more or less of your weight into the client in Chair Massage?

More, Kemo-Sabe

Do I need to say any more?

No Kemo-Sabe ...

〽 〽 〽

Well, actually, I am going to say a little more anyway

I thought you might, Kemo-Sabe

It's just that, with all that I have learnt about the historical accident that led to the almost exclusive development of the use of the hand in Western massage techniques, I was not surprised to see so much harmful use of the hand in Chair Massage

What accident was this, Kemo-Sabe?

The history of bodywork could have gone so many different ways, Tonto

What do you mean, Kemo-Sabe?

Well, Western massage pretty much started out as just a few rubs, a few techniques ...

Even in its medical hey-day in the nineteenth century, Western massage was promoted as a set of techniques for use by the medical profession of the day ...

But Per Henrik Ling's Swedish Massage – this was a therapy, surely?

Yes, it was, Tonto, but it was nothing like the touch therapy that we associate with massage these days.

What was it, Kemo-Sabe?

It was an exercise and stretching therapy much like physiotherapy or movement therapy ...

And massage?

...was literally just one of six strands to this movement therapy – in fact, Ling used to write the massage strokes he wanted performed on his clients as prescriptions

You mean he treated our wondrous and profound therapy as a mere prescription! This I did not know, Kemo-Sabe

Again we need to be careful with our assumptions, Tonto. Just because we are using the word massage does not mean it is the same thing today as two hundred years ago. As I said earlier, bodywork experienced the greatest renaissance that has ever been seen in a therapy

This was in the twentieth century, Kemo-Sabe?

Yes, Tonto. And it is only in the twentieth century that you begin to see massage emerging as an actual therapy in its own right

Why was this, Kemo-Sabe?

Well it is my own opinion that this coincided with a rapidly changing society. This has produced increased stress to the human body and the human psyche

Do you mean the fear of a nuclear holocaust, Kemo-Sabe?

Yes, Tonto, amongst other things. Never before in the history of mankind has there been such an awful possibility – even if we choose not to talk about it

It is always there, Kemo-Sabe

So much so that psychoanalysts are associating it with the emergence of a whole set of neuroses that were unknown prior to the twentieth century

And how does massage fit into this, Kemo-Sabe?

Well, massage provided a flexible system of touch therapy that could respond to these rapidly changing needs of clients

How did this happen, Kemo-Sabe?

Well, by its very nature, massage develops the skill of attunement in the practitioner in a way that is totally unique – I flew through my psychotherapy training because it was always easy for me to attune to the mood shifts in my clients ... something which other psychotherapy students often found hard at first

Yes, Kemo-Sabe – I have found that over the years I have become more sensitive to the psychological as well as to the physical

In my opinion, Tonto, there is no better training for a therapist of any kind than five years working day in and day out with touch and massage

And how did this help massage evolve as a therapy, Kemo-Sabe?

Well, all these sensitised practitioners started to sense the need for different bodywork – for bodywork that could heal the psyche as well as the body

You mean for touch to be more than just a physical or structural therapy, Kemo-Sabe?

Absolutely – the key word here is nurturance

This is what I also believe we are dispensing, when we take our touch out into the marketplace

Yes, I am forever telling therapists to quit marketing themselves as people who give massage and, instead, to start marketing the outcomes that their clients actually achieve

And nurturance is one of these outcomes?

Yes, amongst others

As bodyworkers learn to attune to their clients, their work changes?

Yes. I want to say a little more about this, Tonto, because bodyworkers really need to value the training they are getting whilst they are working – as a training in attunement

And this is something no amount of reading, study or training can give you, Kemo-Sabe!

Yes, it is a wonderful side-effect of a busy practice. It develops attunement and intuition

And you think this intuition is what gives bodyworkers the ability to respond to the needs of clients in a rapidly changing society?

Yes, and along the way invent over a hundred new therapy modalities!

Amazing, Kemo-Sabe

Does that make you feel more excited about your work, Tonto?

Yes, Kemo-Sabe I had no idea that the river of massage had such deep social currents. Lift your saddlebag higher, Kemo-Sabe, or our lunch will get soaked!

Ooops!

You see, Tonto, when I really let myself get excited about this, touch therapy seems to me to be the pre-eminent therapy of the future. We haven't even begun to see the therapeutic explosion in the use of touch as the primary modality of healing that I think will happen over this next century ...

Is that a prediction, Kemo-Sabe?

It most certainly is, Tonto. I believe that the very survival of our species through the twenty-first century will be down to the soothing balm that bodyworkers are offering to our troubled modern psyche

This is a big claim for touch, Kemo-Sabe

Yes it is. Do you agree with it, Tonto?

Yes, I do, Kemo-Sabe, I most assuredly do. Is this something that should go in a

box?

Good idea, Tonto!

> I believe that the very survival of our species through the twenty-first century will be down to the soothing balm that bodyworkers are offering to our troubled modern psyche

Kemo-Sabe?

Yes, Tonto?

I thought we were going to talk about Chair Massage?

Thank you, Tonto I think I just went off on one, didn't I?

You most assuredly did, Kemo-Sabe!

The currents in this river are very strong, Tonto!

Hold your head high, Kemo-Sabe, and take deep breaths!

Okay, so with all this amazing history behind us, this is how it happened that techniques which were only designed for a few minutes' use blossomed into 60-minute therapy sessions ...

Hence the increase in practitioner injury?

Exactly – all because of the way society developed and the tools that practitioners had available. So I have simply expanded the toolbox for practitioners, not so much by teaching techniques as by teaching what I now regard as the seven Postural Secrets to bodywork mastery

This is why I found your NO HANDS Massage so exciting, Kemo-Sabe! The way you teach it gives all the creativity back to the practitioner to apply these Postural Secrets to their own work, whatever style or training they have. But why do you call them secrets, Kemo-Sabe?

Well, whenever I have been privileged to watch or experience the bodywork of true masters, at least five of these ancient Postural Secrets were operational at any one moment, yet no-one seemed to be talking about them

So these secrets are not new, then, Kemo-Sabe?

Absolutely not, they are as old as the mountains, Tonto ...

And as deep as this river, Kemo-Sabe?

Deeper! And now that I teach these Postural Secrets, I am witnessing practitioners evolve into bodywork masters in less than two to three years, whereas it would normally take seven to ten years to develop such mastery

How do you know this, Kemo-Sabe?

Because I have been teaching practitioners for almost twenty years and something different and exciting is now happening

Well, Kemo-Sabe, my own meridian-based bodywork certainly gained a potency and a clarity after learning these seven Postural Secrets ...

And we have come out of the river, Tonto!

Yes, Kemo-Sabe, you did well

Tonto

Yes, Kemo-Sabe?

We are getting close, aren't we?

Yes, Kemo-Sabe, but before we get to the Plateau ...

Where we can learn these seven Postural Secrets ...

And dance with the Dancing Bear, Kemo-Sabe!

Yes, you like that bit, don't you, Tonto?

Kemo-Sabe, it is the most exciting part of the journey and prepares us fully for the summit! But we must stop awhile.

Why?

To dry off in the sun and eat that lunch!

Oh

ꗥ ꗥ ꗥ

So, Kemo-Sabe, have you dried off yet?

Yes, I have, Tonto. That river was a bit scary back there, wasn't it?

Crossing such a raging river is never easy, Kemo-Sabe

So why have we stopped here by this rock face?

We have to climb it, Kemo-Sabe

Climb *that*?

Yes, Kemo-Sabe, I am afraid so

You are joking, of course?

No

I don't suppose there's a way round?

... No, I didn't think you would answer that ... .

Are you ready, Kemo-Sabe? This is a very technical bit of climbing

So we will discuss the technical side of injury prevention on our way up?

Yes, Kemo-Sabe – reach for that crack in the rock, above your head!

Argh! ... so first we need to look at which part of the practitioner's body we are going to use instead of the hands

In order to reduce injury?

Yes. For over ten years, I have been advocating a radical shift in the way we actually deliver our massage strokes

Yes, Kemo-Sabe, I know – put your foot there and rest your fingers for a while

Tonto?

Yes, Kemo-Sabe?

This is going to need some technical skill, isn't it, Tonto?

Yes, Kemo-Sabe, but we will help each other up

And if I fall?

I will hold you with the rope, Kemo-Sabe

Let's get going, then!

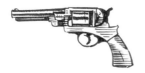

6.
CLIMBING THE ROCKS

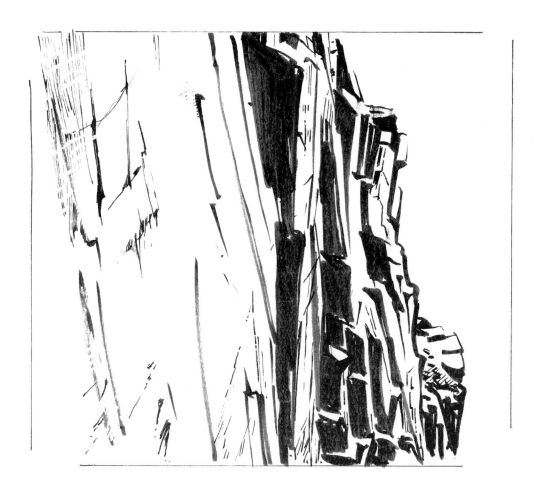

of PODs, four zones, seven surfaces and one soft front

So this technical stuff, Tonto?

Yes, Kemo-Sabe?

It's all about PODs ...

What's a POD, Kemo-Sabe?

It stands for "Point Of Delivery"

And traditionally this has been the hand?

Yes – the whole of Western bodywork literature has been focused on the hand

Until you came along, Kemo-Sabe!

Hi-Yo Silver! Can we have my music here, the tune from the William Tell overture, Tonto?

Kemo-Sabe, they stopped filming us many years ago

Sorry, Tonto, I got carried away ... Where were we?

I was reminding you that, until you publicised this damage to our industry and the solutions of NO HANDS Massage in your first book, there had been a total focus on the hand in our profession's literature

Yes, at last we are seeing the proper use of the forearm being advocated

What do you mean by 'proper' Kemo-Sabe?

Well, for over ten years I have been advocating the use of soft forearm techniques

I have seen sharp and painful forearm techniques being advocated in many different bodywork books

You can spot them a mile off with the clenched fist and the demonic look on the face of the advocates of these horrendous techniques!

They bruise and damage tissues, Kemo-Sabe ...

As well as ensure that the poor recipient will only ever approach bodywork again in moments of sheer desperation!

So we can dismiss these sharp techniques, Kemo-Sabe?

Yes, Tonto, I think we shall just let them fall down to the base of this cliff. Tonto?

Yes, Kemo-Sabe, I know. We are already getting quite high up. Do not look down. Discuss the technical stuff a little more!

Yes, Tonto

Tell me more about PODs, Kemo-Sabe

Well after my own injury, and the discovery of the soft surfaces of the forearm, I realised that the whole body offered many other surfaces with which we could apply our body-weight and pressure to the client's body. So I divided them into four zones

And these zones are, Kemo-Sabe?

Well, if we start with our industry's emphasis on the hand, then we could call anything between the wrist and the tips of your fingers the primary zone

And then by utilising all the different surfaces of the forearm we have created a secondary zone?

Yes, and there are six different surfaces and protuberances suitable for all different types of bodywork – whooooaaaarghhhh!!!!!!

Stop scrabbling, Kemo-Sabe, I have you on the rope

I slipped, Tonto!

I noticed, Kemo-Sabe

And I was just hanging there in the air!

Yes ...

And the rope held ...

That is what it is for, Kemo-Sabe

Thank you, Tonto

You are most welcome. Now you were saying?

Oh yes ... that in the secondary zone of the forearm there are six different surfaces and protuberances suitable for all different types of bodywork

In addition to the soft surface or what you call the soft front?

Yes, this is the really soft part of your forearm very close to your elbow

Just above the medial epicondyle, Kemo-Sabe?

Yes. This is the only forearm surface I teach until my practitioners have had over 6 months of utilising the seven Postural Secrets

Were there any problems using this new approach, Kemo-Sabe?

Yes! My back started to seize up and so did the backs of the people I was sharing my ideas with - we had radically to alter our whole philosophy of movement in order to solve that one!

You say "we", Kemo-Sabe – I thought these ideas were yours?

In the front of my first book I acknowledge some of the practitioners who worked closely with me over the ten years of the development of NO HANDS Massage. And there were many others who I could not even mention because of space ...

How did you spend ten years with them, Kemo-Sabe?

Well, by running monthly professional development groups

This was more than just practical training, then?

Oh yes, there is so much more that affects the success of a practitioner than just practical skill

And in these monthly groups you would teach your NO HANDS ideas?

There was no way I could avoid it – these practitioners dragged them out of me!

And then?

Well, then they went away and tried them out on all *their* clients.

How many practitioners was this, Kemo-Sabe?

Well at my most busy, I was running four of these groups every month, each group having about eight to ten practitioners. Over the ten years a conservative estimate would be two groups a month

And how many clients did these practitioners see?

Well, they probably averaged about ten clients each a week

Kemo-Sabe, are you telling me that these ideas were tried out on almost 200 clients a week for over ten years?

Yes, that is quite a lot, isn't it, Tonto?

That's over 100,000 massages, Kemo-Sabe!

That many?

And each month they would come back and discuss these new techniques with you?

Yes, and this gave me the opportunity to correct any mistakes they were making. Sometimes I would have to refine the strokes a bit further. It's where I learnt how to teach this stuff to practitioners

A sort of stroke laboratory?

Yes! And we formulated three criteria for the adoption of each new technique

What were they, Kemo-Sabe?

Well, the first was obviously that the new techniques we were formulating should be zero strain ... Aaaaaarrgghhhhh!

Hold tight! That was much better, Kemo-Sabe – can you grab that ledge?

Yep ... I slipped again, Tonto

I noticed

Thank you again, Tonto

You are most welcome, Kemo-Sabe

🌿 🌿 🌿

So the first of your criterion for strokes was that they should be zero strain - for the practitioners, Kemo-Sabe?

Yes

And your second criteria, Kemo-Sabe?

Well, the second of our criteria was that the stroke should be more effective than the one it replaced ...

For the client?

Yes, Tonto

And the third?

The third of our criteria was that each of these new strokes should actually do something to improve the health of the practitioner as well as the client

This is your "healing synergy" principle, Kemo-Sabe?

Well this is the principle behind all seven Postural Secrets

It is the principle that binds all your work into a coherent whole Kemo-Sabe?

I suppose it is, Tonto – yes, I had never thought of it like that until now – Thank you, Tonto

You are most welcome, Kemo-Sabe.

ᘐ ᘐ ᘐ

Kemo-Sabe?

Yes, Tonto?

We were discussing the Four Zones

Yes, so after I discovered that the forearm had many soft surfaces ...

As well as sharp ones, Kemo-Sabe!

Which only my master practitioners are shown how to use properly and safely ...

After this secondary zone, Kemo-Sabe?

Well, I found myself beginning to use parts of my upper arm ...

And this you called the tertiary zone?

And then anything from the shoulder joint to the tip of our heads and the tips of our toes became the quarterly zone

And the value of these distinctions?

Well, simply that bodywork literature has never written about massage in this way before, Tonto

There is an assumption that only the primary zone is worth writing about and teaching?

Yes, and I regard this as a mistake

But Kemo-Sabe, surely the focus on the primary zone is based on the profession's need for dexterity and sensitivity?

It is true that the hand is clearly the most dextrous part of the body, and provides the best surface for subtle palpation. However, this does not justify its exclusivity, in my opinion

And what's more, Tonto, the vast majority of massage techniques require neither complex dexterity nor palmar sensitivity. Now we can protect the hand ...

To do the sensitive work even better, Kemo-Sabe?

Exactly. I am a passionate protector of the sensitive hand

So your intention is to help preserve the hands and backs of as many practitioners of this creative profession as possible, Kemo-Sabe?

Yes. The use of other parts of the body ensures that the hands are protected precisely so that they can be used for what they are best at – namely, dexterity and sensitivity.

This seems very logical, Kemo-Sabe. But some practitioners think that we need to do deep structural work that involves the tiring use of hands and fingers. Have you noticed how the number of books on these structural aspects outnumber books on the energetic, emotional, mental and even the spiritual effects of massage?

Yes, I have, Tonto, but this does not necessarily reflect the public's interest

Well, Kemo-Sabe, people often complain of a stiff or aching shoulder, but what they are really coming for is deep relaxation

Precisely, Tonto. The experience of massage practitioners is that clients are looking for all sorts of different outcomes, including nurturance

And simply learning more structural techniques is not necessarily going to help the practitioner deal with their clients

A basic level of structural skill is required. However, what is often missed is that one of the best ways to deal with structural problems anywhere in the body is with "systemic bodywork"

What do you mean by "systemic bodywork"?

I mean bodywork that is done in such a way that the whole body relaxes and softens and melts, regardless of where the practitioner is working or which techniques are being employed ... .

Now this every bodyworker knows, Kemo-Sabe: when the client just sinks into the Chair and lets out a great big sigh of release!

Yes, that's it, Tonto. And sometimes this is just from taking the time to lean in

r e e e e e e e a l s l o w

Yet this is barely mentioned in most books or manuals, Kemo-Sabe!

As I have said, Tonto, much bodywork that has been written and taught has been heavily influenced by bodywork structuralists

And you are not a structuralist, Kemo-Sabe?

Well, like most bodyworkers I built my clinic on my structural effectiveness – but not by using structural techniques

Instead, you used "systemic bodywork"?

Exactly! If anything, you could call me a "systemist"!

I think I will stick to Kemo-Sabe, Kemo-Sabe

You see, Tonto, if we use the analogy of clothing, the aches and pains clients actually show us are places where the fabric has torn, whereas the reason for tearing is that the material has shrunk. What most clients present us with is one goddam shrunken suit, and what they need is a new,

s t r e t c h y suit,

rather than just having the tear mended

Which means it will simply tear all over again!

Yes! You see, NO HANDS Massage does this systemic work particularly well. On a physical level practitioners want to be effective in loosening and stretching the suit. And once the suit is stretched, the client's own body often sorts itself out and restructures itself ...

Back into a more balanced postural configuration of muscle, tendon, ligament and bone, Kemo-Sabe ...

And mind and soul, Tonto

Of course, Kemo-Sabe. And much of this systemic work does not need the dexterity of the hand?

You've got it, Tonto.

What about the argument that the hand is gentle and conveys a reassuring human contact ?

Well, this is exactly my points, soft and gentle touch does not need to be replaced, as this gives no stress to the practitioner's joints. When reassurance and nurturance are required, then, by definition, there is *no harm* to the practitioner's palmar surface, fingers or wrists taking place ...

And no need for the abandonment of the hands

Just so. In actual fact, many other surfaces of the practitioner's body can provide this reassurance, if applied with awareness

So the forearm can reassure as effectively as the hand?

Yes, Tonto, and not only the forearm ... and what is more important, after more than ten years of teaching NO HANDS Massage, I have yet to find a conventional massage technique, manipulation or stretch that cannot be replaced by the creative and sensitive use of other parts of the practitioner's body

This is what this book is all about, Kemo-Sabe

Yes, we want to share some of these alternatives

It was very exciting to find that many Chair Massage techniques were actually improved upon through the creative application of forearm techniques

Yes, and it is important to stress that this statement is based on the comments of practitioners and clients

And, Kemo-Sabe, equally important is the fact that students report a surge of excitement and renewed interest in their work due to the whole body creativity which is required when the hands are abandoned

Yes, the seven Postural Secrets stimulate the practitioner's natural creativity. Tonto!

Kemo-Sabe?

We are at the Plateau of the Bear!

Yes, Kemo-Sabe

That was brilliant – once I got into a rhythm

You did not do badly – for a white man

Thank you, Tonto

So now, are we ready to move onto these seven Postural Secrets, Kemo-Sabe?

So we can do the Dancing Bear, Tonto? Have we finished all our technical stuff?

Yes, Kemo-Sabe. We have finished with all our PODs and have now reached the home of the Dancing Bear

So it is time to dance?

Yes, Kemo-Sabe, most assuredly yes!

Then let us meet the Bear!

Let us go quickly, Kemo-Sabe, for in all things, timing is everything!

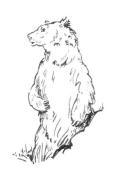

7. On the Plateau
of the
DANCING
BEAR

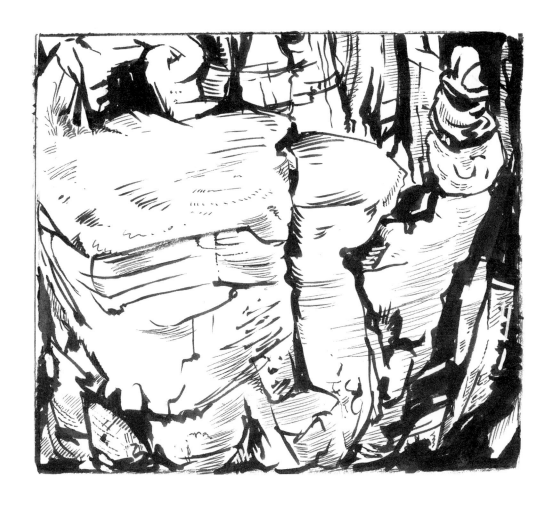

1. The Power of *Hara*

So first, we must ...

Begin in the belly, Kemo-Sabe?

Yes, I believe that all massage strokes begin energetically in the practitioner's belly. This is also called the "*Hara*" in oriental literature.

Did you know, Kemo-Sabe, that in experiments on athletes they discovered that before any skeletal muscles in the legs or arms contract, there is a contraction in the belly that can be measured electronically?

So science is finally catching up with the ancient masters of bodywork!

Yes, Kemo-Sabe, and if you stand in a room with your eyes closed, you can feel this "pre-movement" going on in the Hara if you really breathe and slow down and imagine you are massaging someone in the air ...

"Air massage", Tonto – like playing "air guitar"?

Most assuredly, Kemo-Sabe!

I think we need a "Do It Now" box, don't you, Tonto?

Yes, Kemo-Sabe. And our practitioners need to know that if they read on without doing these exercises then they will be missing the best bit!

So the "Do It Now" Box means just that – DO NOT READ ON UNDER ANY CIRCUMSTANCES ... until you have actually "done it"!

Shall I tell them, Kemo-Sabe?

Go on, then

Well, if you start your day with what is in this chapter your bodywork...

And your Life, Tonto!

Yes, your bodywork and your life WILL NEVER BE THE SAME AGAIN ...

Stand in the middle of the room and take a few moments to connect with your breath and with your whole body.

With each breath, increase your awareness of the sensations in your body...

Now, start to do a massage stroke in front of you – concentrate only on the first quarter of the stroke and take 4 times longer than usual to make that first part of the stroke ...

Feel what happens in your belly ... *just before your arms start to move ...*

If you don't feel any pre-movement in your belly, *slow down* and concentrate on what happens *just before you actually move*

Between the idea and the actual movement...

... An impulse in your belly

So if you did not feel this, do not worry. It just means you need to do it lots and lots more

　　　　　　　　and breathe and move and

　　　　　　　　　　　　think from your belly more ...

So, Kemo-Sabe, before anything actually moves there is an impulse, an activation towards movement, a stirring in the belly?

Yes, according to *Shiatsu* principles, practically all our meridians and energy lines emanate outwards from this centre, radiating out to the limbs and returning back again

Yes, Kemo-Sabe, the great masters of Shiatsu can diagnose and treat the energy imbalances of the whole body through the belly

This is because the *Hara* is the place from which we drew our nourishment and our life force in the womb. The *Hara* is the place into which we breathe and from which we breathe out. As the seat of this life force, Buddha figures are shown with wonderfully rounded bellies ...

Unlike our modern day fetish about trim torsos, Kemo-Sabe?

Yes, Tonto, a large belly like yours was regarded as a sign of wisdom and power in oriental art and literature

I knew there was a reason it was so hard to reduce! So how do we grow and develop our power in this Hara, Kemo-Sabe?

By doing these *Hara* exercises over and over.

I think we need another box which is a "Do It Often" box, Kemo-Sabe

Yes, Tonto

DO IT OFTEN

——————

Stand in the middle of the room with your legs slightly apart and your knees bent. Place your hands on your belly. Feel your breath entering and leaving your belly. Let your belly expand with each in-breath, and collapse with each out-breath. Close your eyes as you do this. Open up your awareness to all the physical sensations of your standing and your breathing. Make this the centre of your focus: your belly, your breath and your connect-edness

---

As bodyworkers, we want to let each stroke emanate from the belly?

Exactly so, Tonto

How long should we concentrate on this one before moving onto the next Postural Secret, Kemo-Sabe ?

I should think a couple of hundred years should just about do it justice, Tonto

Is that all, Kemo-Sabe?!

2. Some *sole* secrets

So what happens after the beginning, Kemo-Sabe? What happens after we feel this impulse, this energetic beginning in our Hara, what happens next?

Well, Tonto, movement happens. But the really important question is *how* the movement happens

Well, in the case of a massage movement, my whole body moves, Kemo-Sabe ...

Ah, but which part moves first? Where does the stroke truly begin?

I am not sure, Kemo-Sabe – my legs, my hips?

All those do move, Tonto – but not at first!

Mmmm ... this is a hard question, Kemo-Sabe!

Yes, it is! But wouldn't it be worth knowing where each stroke truly has its birth?

Yes, Kemo-Sabe, if we could know this much about our strokes then our movements would surely be powerful and precise because of this awareness

People often ask me whether I had dance training – and the truth is I haven't been to a single dance class in my entire life ... but I believe that if anything has helped my movements to be graceful it is this awareness of where movement actually begins, Tonto

Of where the stroke begins?

Yes, where it begins its life – what happens in the belly is like a *conception*, but the movement takes its actual physical *birth* or manifestation from the place of its beginning ... I asked myself this question during every stroke of every massage for over three years, Tonto

And what did you find?

Well, I found that just before the whole body moves and after the impulse to movement from the belly there is a dropping of energy into the ground, INTO *the feet* ...

What you mean, Kemo-Sabe?

To make any movement. including massage strokes, we have to push down against the earth

Yes, Kemo-Sabe, we have known for a long time that the rutting wild boar has to push down on the earth in order to stick his horns up the behind of the of the wandering gold prospector ...

Tonto, you promised me ...

No more rutting, Kemo-Sabe?

No more rutting, Tonto

Sorry, Kemo-Sabe

So this means that the first part of our body to experience pressure and force is the *sole* of the foot against the earth

So it's all in the "sole", Kemo-Sabe?

Sole Secrets, Tonto, or...

Secrets of the Soul!

Yes, Tonto, I believe the secrets of *all massage* may actually lie in the sole of the foot, which is why I spend so much time emphasising *sole*

When we focus on our physical sensations we can actually feel it going like this ...

The movement has its *energetic* beginning in the belly...

Then we feel a sudden and rapid *earthing of energy* ...

This is observed as a *postural sinking* prior to any stroke beginning ...

Without this *anchoring,* our movements lack potency or power ...

And with it, Kemo-Sabe?

With it, we are friends with the source of our power – the earth. Without the strong earth to push against we would be flailing impotently around in space, no matter how physically strong we were ...

So bodywork power is in our connection with the earth and not in our muscles?

Absolutely! By allowing our whole bodyweight to drop down into the feet, by keeping our awareness in our feet, we stay grounded in our movements and at the same time increase our potency as practitioners. In this way, attaining good posture is not only about looking after ourselves ...

But also about becoming more effective, Kemo-Sabe!

Exactly, so we approach each stroke energetically from the *Hara,* and then allow it to drop down into our feet. This is accompanied by an actual physical lowering of our stance.

So this is why it is so important to feel all of our movements through the soles of our feet?

Yes, Tonto – in fact, we have discovered that it is almost impossible to make *any* movement in your body that cannot be felt in your feet

And this way practitioners stay focused on the source of their strength and power through the soles of their feet. So how do practitioners develop these Sole Secrets?

I think we need a "Do It Now" Box

DO IT NOW

Stand in the middle of the room, legs apart, keeping your knees bent, breathing into your belly. Do this for several breaths. Now let the weight of your belly drop down into your feet. Do this by letting your lower back lengthen, tucking your pelvis slightly under. Accompany this with a slight lowering of your knees. Make this a very small movement. Make sure your upper body stays upright and your chest nice and open and wide. Focus your mind's attention on the soles of your feet. Can you feel this *dropping down* in your feet?

Make small movements with your arms or your hips and notice how each movement is experienced in the soles of your feet. By moving your belly and torso slowly, you can feel the different reflex zones of your feet becoming activated. Imagine that the earth is actually massaging your feet through the floor. This is a pleasant rebalancing exercise that you can do almost anywhere at any time. Do this for as long as you wish - even a minute will be beneficial, and 5-10 minutes will awaken and energise all the reflexes in your feet for the rest of the day

And when we are massaging, Kemo-Sabe?

Aways feel your movements in your feet – I focused my awareness for three years on just this *one thing* and at the end I realised that my bodywork had taken a quantum leap in its power and its potency...

So we focus on the feet, Kemo-Sabe?

Yes, Tonto, until you can touch the very "Sole" of bodywork

DO IT OFTEN

⟫⟩-◊-⟨⟪

Whatever you are doing – always feel your movements in your feet. Feel every action you make having its physical beginning in the **soles** of your feet

3. It's all in the *flow*

What is the third Postural Secret, Kemo-Sabe?

> It is the secret of water, Tonto

Ah, this is the principle of "flow"?

> Yes, to really grasp the power of *flow* we need to abandon all ideas of correct or incorrect posture

And only see movement?

> Yes. The problem with most bodywork posture as I see it is the problem of trying to capture it in static drawings or photographs …

I love these drawings in your books, Kemo-Sabe – because they seem to capture such movement

> Yes, Tonto, and John Coombes has been drawing dancers for many, many years, so he was the perfect person to capture the flow in bodywork. The danger is that rigid angular images are likely to produce rigid body movements in the practitioner. What we need instead are more *poetic* ways of drawing, writing and describing posture

We need poetry, Kemo-Sabe?

> Yes, I find that the use of the dynamic language of primal and elemental imagery is helpful in capturing what I believe are the core principles of bodywork posture

Yes, Kemo-Sabe, so far, we have been using the elemental language and imagery of the earth and words such as rooted, anchored and grounded to convey the Postural Secrets of Hara and sole

> And for this third Postural Secret, we need to hold in our minds the dynamic image conjured up by the word "flow". To evoke this Postural Secret, I encourage practitioners to think in terms of the element water and the concept of whole body flow

78

And, Kemo-Sabe, this is this true even for the still moments in bodywork?

> Even more so, for when the practitioner is totally still, sometimes it is only then that the full flow of the life-force within the client's body can be truly felt

And how do we develop this sense of flow, Kemo-Sabe?

> Well, by treating your whole session as consisting of *one stroke*

One massage stroke per session?

> Yes, so all your movements quite literally *flow* into each other

Can we practise this now Kemo-Sabe?

> Well, we won't learn to dance with the Bear by just reading about all this, will we?

Most certainly not, Kemo-Sabe!

DO IT NOW

Put on a piece of serene, tranquil, flowing music.

Stand in the middle of the room, with knees bent and eyes shut.

Activate your awareness of your breath, your belly and your feet.

Gently sway from side to side, and then forwards and backwards.

Let your arms enter into this swaying and flowing.

Let the sound of your breath be part of this ebbing and flowing movement.

Do this for the next three years ...

So, Kemo-Sabe, if we hold such flowing elemental images in our minds during bodywork sessions, then we are less likely to damage our bodies?

> Yes, because there is no rigidity to cause strain. Nothing is held long enough to cause any strain or injury ...

Effortless flow, like great rivers flowing though the land ...

> Yes, Tonto, this is the most powerful bodywork

We cut through tension and muscle tightness like the great rivers cutting through rock ...

> Ah, Tonto, that is beautiful. Sometimes you just blow me away ...

Massage as dance, Kemo-Sabe!

Yes, Tonto. Massage as dance. The human bodyworker is a dancer who is in continuous movement, creating physical poetry

To watch such a bodyworker is to be mesmerised by flow and movement and by the beauty and grace of such bodywork ...

Yes, Tonto, it is the most beautiful sight in the world ...

DO IT OFTEN

Now visualise being in your massage room, giving a *one-stroke session* so that all your movements flow into each other.

Imagine yourself slowly moving around the table and massaging your client ...

Feel all your movements flow from your belly, down into your feet and then feel them *flow* through your legs into *movement*

Let your whole body become the flowing element of water

---

4. The art of falling

And the fourth Postural Secret, Kemo-Sabe?

This one eliminates all possibility of back strain, because it is the secret of falling-over massage

Now, Kemo-Sabe, this is the most outrageous thought – literally to "fall" onto our clients

Yes, whether the client is in a chair or on a table we can let the client support us totally

Wasn't this the first one you discovered?

Yes, in despair at my second wrist injury within three hours I "flipped out" mentally and found myself totally slumped on my client's back ...

And he was making positive sounds?

Yes, he was purring with the pleasure that my bodyweight was causing as his muscles stretched and compressed ...

But there is more to this "falling" than just falling onto our clients, surely, Kemo-Sabe?

Yes, in most cases if we just fell onto our clients we would be out of business in no time – it is actually about a controlled collapse through transferring bodyweight

So we start with all our bodyweight in our feet?

Yes, and then we slowly transfer our weight into the client's body through our arms ...

Until all our weight is supported by the client

And we have *zero strain* in our back. This is what we do with NO HANDS Massage: we lean on our client by falling gracefully onto them – more of a *lean* than a push.

If we literally fell onto our clients, Kemo-Sabe, then this would cause them pain!

Yes, it is more of a slow motion *transfer* of our weight from the ground onto our client

To understand this I actually had to change the way I thought about my own movements, Kemo-Sabe: no longer do I think of myself as standing or walking, but as crawling ...

Yes, Tonto, because most bodywork involves the distribution of our weight between four points: two feet and two arms and hands

Just like crawling! So we need to practice transferring our weight from one to the other

Yes, transferring our weight from the feet, onto the arms and hands and vice-versa

Can we do this now, Kemo-Sabe?

Yup!

Stand facing a wall, and place your forearms lightly, at chest height, against the wall with all your weight going down into your feet

You are now self-supporting

Now, bend your knees and *very slowly* lean into the wall.

Feel your arms filling with your bodyweight and beginning to press against the wall.

As your weight transfers into your arms there is an increase of pressure against the wall

Now, tuck your hips under, bend your knees and let the weight *slowly* empty out of your arms and back into your legs.

See how slowly you can do this and how subtle the transfer of weight can feel.

Move further away from the wall, or closer in, to experiment with transferring different amounts of body weight

This concept has really helped me to eliminate any back pain from giving bodywork, Kemo-Sabe

Well, that is because all back strain comes from leaning forward and holding ourselves from falling. There is no need to do this in NO HANDS Massage

Because it is now safe to fall?

Yes

The end of all back strain – this is a good thing, Kemo-Sabe?

Yup

DO IT OFTEN

—⟫•⟪—

Whenever you are between massage sessions, stand close to the table with a large pile of pillows in front of you.

Begin with all your bodyweight in your feet so that your hands and arms are resting with only their own weight on the pillows. Put all your body weight into your heels.

Now, rock forward onto the balls of your feet and *slowly* feel your weight entering and *filling* your arms

And then rock back into your heels again *slowly*

Note how the slow transfer of your weight from legs to arms changes the height of your pillows

Do this many times over until you can identify the exact percentage of your bodyweight that is in your arms and feet respectively

5. Resting on the Pillars of Support

So, Kemo-Sabe, we have Hara ...

And *sole* ...

And flow ...

And *falling* ...

What is the fifth Postural Secret, Kemo-Sabe?

Well, Tonto, the fifth is *support*. It is the secret that surrounds us all in our lives, but which we often fail to appreciate or enjoy

This one I really liked, Kemo-Sabe, because it gave me permission to look at my work as surrounded by support

Yes, Tonto, this one starts with the premise that all bodywork should be as comfortable as possible – indeed, the principle of falling has *support* embedded deep within it

Because with falling, the client physically supports the practitioner's weight?

Yes. And *support* is about seeking out all the places during a massage that can give physical support to us - both from the chair and from the client

But, Kemo-Sabe, I was taught not to bump into the table or the chair during a session!

Yes, I know. Yet there is nothing intrinsically unethical about using the table or the chair to lean on and get support ...

And leaning on the client?

Well, if we are leaning on the client for the purposes of giving bodywork, then our weight is the stroke

Then support is simply how we deliver the stroke

Well actually there is more to support than just how we deliver each stroke. We get support from our very attitude and use of the table and the client – even from the air molecules that surround us.

And this is the principle of *support* Tonto – to regard the very molecules around us as holding us up and supporting us during massage

It is about how we see ourselves, Kemo-Sabe

It is both about how we see ourselves, and it is also about the specific nuts and bolts of how we actually move, what we lean on and what we use for physical support during the massage. To do this we need to understand both the use of *secret levers* and *triangulation*?

What are these secret levers, Kemo-Sabe?

Secret levers are all the little supports that surround us during bodywork that most practitioners ignore

Like the edge of a table or the leg of a chair?

Or the shoulder that invitingly suggests itself as a leaning post while I massage down the back

And triangulation, Kemo-Sabe?

With *triangulation* we always think of creating triangles of support between ourselves, the chair and the client's body. The triangle is an amazing geometrical shape and the strongest known to mankind – it was used to build the first bridges – in bodywork the outside triangle is from the floor where the practitioner's feet are ...

To the top of the practitioner's body ...

And down though the client's body, the chair and back into the floor ...

Which holds a tension back to the practitioner's feet?

Yes, through the floorboards

I like this idea of the floor holding the tension very much, Kemo-Sabe

So the practitioner can relax. We always aim to look like the *laziest* bodyworkers in the world, Tonto, so that through this ancient Postural Secret of *support* the massage session becomes a time of healing for the practitioner as well as the client – healing synergy, in fact

Is this where 1 + 1 = 3 Kemo-Sabe?

Yes, where the practitioner gives (1) and the client receives (1) and then the magical bit is that the practitioner also receives (1 again). This is why one plus actually equals three!

So the practitioner receives the healing benefits from the massage as well as the client. I like this 1 + 1 = 3 very much! I always knew my maths teachers did not see the whole picture, Kemo-Sabe!

Can we have a "Do It Now" box, Kemo-Sabe?

Yup

DO IT NOW

Stand close to a wall, side on, so that one shoulder is closer to the wall and one is further away

Lean into this wall

Feel your weight falling into two ends of the triangle, your shoulder leaning into the top apex of the triangle and your feet into the bottom corner of the triangle

Feel the tension in the floor as it stops your feet from sliding away from the wall

Picture this triangle of support and *relax* as many of your muscles as possible

After a few minutes, swap shoulders and repeat

This is good, Kemo-Sabe – it is amazing how much tension I can release with such a simple exercise

Yes, it is surprisingly powerful

---

6. A proposal for kneeling

The sixth Postural Secret actually follows on nicely from this one about support, because it is all about *kneeling*

With a cushion under the knee I hope, Kemo-Sabe

Yes, or a nice thick carpet will often suffice

Why is kneeling so important, Kemo-Sabe?

Well, as I said earlier, Tonto, unless we are actually *falling* onto the client, our own back is experiencing strain every time we lean forward …

And kneeling means we can do bodywork that is powerful because we can keep our back vertical?

Yes, while powering our movements from the *hips* so that the hips become the powerhouse of all our movements

But Kemo-Sabe – how can we reach all the body if we are kneeling?

Well, there are many parts of a Chair Massage that are quite low down. So we are either *falling* or *kneeling*

Show me this kneeling, Kemo-Sabe

A "Do It Now" box?

Most assuredly, Kemo-Sabe

DO IT NOW

—▸◦◂—

With a pillow under your knee take up what I call "'The Proposal Stance" with one knee on the floor and one foot on the floor

Practice lunging towards your forward upright knee – keeping your spine *vertical*

Experience the amount of travelling that you do as you stretch your groin in the forwards movement

Imagine transferring that amount of movement into your client's body as a massage stroke, all the time keeping your back totally *strain-free*

Kemo-Sabe?

Yes, Tonto?

I understand how this helps with a table – but how does it make a difference with a chair?

There are many parts of the client's body that we can massage far more effectively from this kneeling position. Even within your Kata there are places - for the lower back moves that we perform on the chair – where applying pressure this low down can be tiring for the practitioner; with *kneeling* it is a pleasure and almost a rest

Is this your "resting while running", Kemo-Sabe?

Yes. In fell running we learn psychologically to rest while going downhill: even though it looks like we are running, we are actually letting the gradient do the running and we just relax into falling down a hill

And in kneeling?

Well, we can use it to take a breather during the session

This is important if we are seeing a lot of clients one after the other?

Yes, Tonto – this Postural Secret turns us into marathon runners ...

We can just keep on going?

Because of the ease and efficiency of all our movements

So this is worth a lot of money, Kemo-Sabe?

This Postural Secret alone enables bodyworkers to earn hundreds of thousands of pounds, Tonto ...

By enabling us to see more clients for more years with less effort!

Yes, so that our careers can lengthen, our learning deepen and our wisdom and effectiveness as practitioners increase

That is exactly the sort of bodywork equation I like to hear, Kemo-Sabe!

<hr />

7. About gazelles, ploughing and the shire horse

So, Kemo-Sabe, what is the seventh Postural Secret?

Well this one is all about gazelles and shire horses

You mean we use the shire horse for the really heavy work?

Yes, like in ploughing, and we protect the graceful gazelle for all the delicate work

How does this work in practice Kemo-Sabe?

Well, in terms of Points Of Delivery the shire horse is the soft front

And the gazelle is the hand?

Yes.

There is more?

Yes, it is also about *vectoring* - the split second before we lean into a stroke we check to see that our body is aligned fully behind the intended direction of the stroke

And sometimes this means actually stopping and moving my body to a different position entirely before beginning the stroke?

Yes. So, for example, if I am wanting to press into the shoulder, I need to be clear in which direction I intend to push the tissues. Then I check to see that my whole body is aligned behind the stroke ...

Often by actually repositioning our legs, Kemo-Sabe?

Yes, amongst other more subtle adjustments

I feel the power of this when I use it, Kemo-Sabe, but how does this happen?

Well, the tension in the client's body is important – it has often taken months, sometimes years, and often involves some very big muscles

Muscles that are much bigger than the tiny muscles between a practitioner's fingers and thumbs

Exactly, and sometimes these big tight muscles in our clients will soften like putty if they are faced by such an array of weight and power

So the bodywork is a war and a pushing contest?

No, quite the reverse. With the shire horse as my guiding Postural Secret I find my work actually gets softer and gentler

You mean the muscle tension just surrenders?

Yes, as the client's body senses the *potential* power and strength that is possible behind the stroke

It just melts, Kemo-Sabe?

Experienced masters of bodywork hardly ever use force, Tonto. They quietly and gently *enquire* as to whether the body really wants to struggle before letting go ...

Effortlessly and painlessly

Exactly. Shall we have a 'Do It Now' box, Tonto?

Most assuredly, Kemo-Sabe

DO IT NOW

Facing straight at a wall, lean against the wall on your forearms

Place your legs a good distance away from the wall so you have a good triangle

Place one foot forward – for control and just imagine the *line of power* that runs from your feet through your whole body into the wall

Imagine that, if you kept up this *line of power* for long enough, the wall would eventually give way and crumble – this is *shire horse*

Now take your hips to one side, and feel the *loss* of pressure and power against the wall

This is what working without the *shire horse* is about

Now go back and feel the power of leaning your whole body *in one direction* again

---

And all of this can be achieved in the moment before we lean, Kemo-Sabe?

Yes, although sometimes it means not making the stroke we were about to make, and instead we pause ... and spend time working out what we want to achieve and then align the body to create the desired *vectors of force*

If necessary, going from our arms back down to our feet?

Yes, and only then, when we are properly aligned from head to toe, do we actually lean into our client

To be on the receiving end of such focused leaning is truly powerful, Kemo-Sabe

Yes it is, Tonto..

And you have an equation for all this shire horse work?

Yes, it is simply that the strength and weight of the practitioner's applied force must be greater than the muscle resistance of the client, even if we do not use it all; which can be translated into the following equation:

$$S = P > C$$

where S = Successful practice, P = Practitioner weight and strength and C = Client's tensile muscle strength

So in every session and with every movement we make, we must ask ourselves whether we have got this equation right, Kemo-Sabe?

Yup

Which bring us to …

Dances with Bears

This is what I have been waiting for, Kemo-Sabe! Can we do it now?

Yes, as a celebration of all the travelling and learning that we have done together, Tonto. I think it is time to be outrageous and take the big grizzly's fat paw

And to stare into his great big ugly muzzle, Kemo-Sabe!

And learn the steps of

Of his crazy mad dance, Kemo-Sabe!

Yes, Tonto, this has been what the journey has all been for – to learn the Dance of the Dancing Bear

So this bit is more important than anything else?

This bit is the whole book – this is the bit we most need to get to the Summit, Tonto.

Look at how far we had to travel to get here.

So if you have travelled this far with us, reader …

They are all here with us now, Kemo-Sabe

Then you will appreciate the value of moving in a way that embodies all seven of the Postural Secrets.

In other words, Dancing with the Bear!

So, before we even look at the new strokes we are going to use on the Chair …

We do the important part right here …

Right now

Let's do it, Kemo-Sabe

We have no choice Tonto – look!

Yes Kemo-Sabe

The Great Bear is here …

DOING THE BEAR

—➤-◆-◄—

Stand in the middle of the room

Let your knees and arms bend

Breathe into your belly and drop your weight into the floor

'Flop' your jaw open

'Flop' your wrists

Let your head fall forward so it too can 'flop'

Now, move around the room like a bear

Feel like a bear

Become a Dancing Bear

Congratulations! You are now ...

... *"Doing the Bear"*

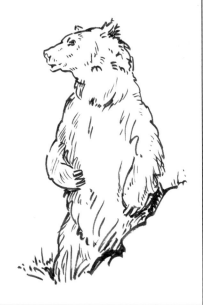

Oh, Kemo-Sabe – this is the best of all – I feel so powerful and relaxed when I do this!

That, Tonto, is the very essence of NO HANDS Massage.

When I sees practitioner *Doing the Bear* in their work or in their everyday movements I just know they have really got it – and what powerful bodywork they must be giving to their clients!

Oooooh! Say that again, Kemo-Sabe!

In a box, Tonto?

Most assuredly, Kemo-Sabe

When I see a practitioners *Doing the Bear* in their work or in their everyday movements, I just know they have really got it – and what powerful bodywork they must be giving to their clients

---

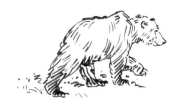

8. Pausing on a ledge

JUST BELOW THE SUMMIT

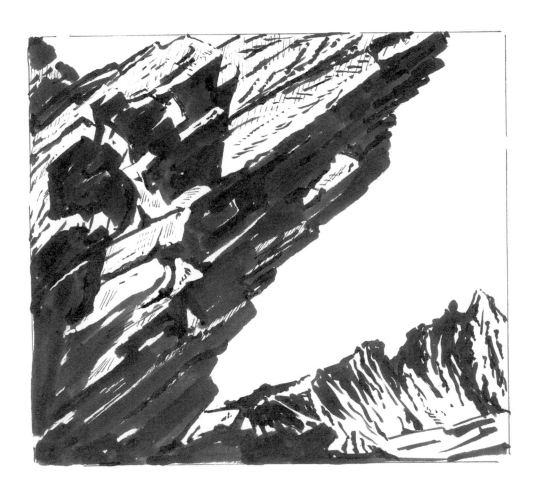

Kemo-Sabe?

Yes, Tonto?

That was wonderful!

Yes – it is something else to lose oneself in *the Bear*, isn't it?

Can we do this during our sessions, Kemo-Sabe?

It is a requirement, Tonto ...

Because?

Out of this posture, which summarises everything we have learned along the way, comes all the bodywork wisdom I have ever learned.

Tell me more about this, Kemo-Sabe

Well, Tonto, it's a physical knowing, something that only happens when we lose ourselves so completely in the "now" of our bodywork. Sometimes, it feels as if centuries may have passed by the time the session is over, and in this altered state it almost feels as if the bodywork is guiding me, rather than the other way round ...

Ah, this is the moment when the Great Spirit of massage takes over the session!

Well, yes, you could say that ...

I have felt this wondrous feeling, Kemo-Sabe

Because you are one of the best, Tonto

And you think doing the Bear is the key to this feeling?

Yes. *Doing the Bear* is the postural nuts and bolts of this profound bodywork concept, whether you are working for ten minutes or sixty

This is a very spiritual part of bodywork, isn't it, Kemo-Sabe?

It is the very heart of it

ℓ ℓ ℓ

Kemo-Sabe?

Yes, Tonto?

Before we finally climb to the top of the mountain, can we summarise all we have seen and done?

Are we that close, Tonto?

Yes, Kemo-Sabe – we have travelled a long time together, and it is not far now

So it is a great idea to look back over our journey, because what people actually see of NO HANDS Massage, is just people standing on the Summit. They do not see how many supplies we had to take with us or how far we had to travel even to reach the base of this mountain

It has been a fun journey so far, Kemo-Sabe

Yes, it has, hasn't it, Tonto … so where did we start?

Well, Kemo-Sabe, first in our journey we had to cross that Boggy Marshland

Yes, Tonto, we did, didn't we? And you taught me how to walk lightly through the mire, where as many as 78 per cent of all practitioners could be getting injured

That was a bad place, Kemo-Sabe

And then we climbed the Foothills of Chair Massage History in order to see how it all began …

How it evolved mainly from acupressure or anma techniques

Yes and we met some very impressive practitioners

Oh yes, Kemo-Sabe, people working in cancer wards and in hospitals and doing powerful research – I liked meeting Ruaring Massage Brave and Petrissage Pete …

And then, do you remember the dark Ravine where we had to discover a new language for describing bodywork accurately?

Yes, Kemo-Sabe, and we came out with a clear definition of two different types of Chair Massage:

Muscle-based for Western approaches

And meridian-based for Oriental approaches

So, by holding onto the linguistic accuracy of meridian-based bodywork and muscle-based bodywork we got through the Ravine – just!

And then we had to cross that deep and fast-flowing River, Kemo-Sabe

Yes, of course! I remember now, where we looked at the historical development of our profession's dependency or even obsession with, the hand.

And how massage has changed so much

And how massage practitioners, as purveyors of touch, have been able to meet the growing needs for our society for mental as well as physical soothing

And then there was that difficult Rock Face we had to climb, Kemo-Sabe

Yes, and all that talk about the technical aspects of NO HANDS Massage …

The PODs Kemo-Sabe!

Yes, and the Four Zones

And then we climbed onto the Plateau of The Dancing Bear

Where we learned how the seven Postural Secrets to bodywork mastery are more important than any actual techniques

That NO HANDS Massage is all about principles rather than techniques

Yes, Tonto – all experienced bodyworkers discover that techniques are just for nervous and inexperienced beginners

And these Postural Secrets go to the very soul of massage!

> Yes, and if we break this down scientifically, we can say that masterful bodyworkers begin each stroke in the belly ...

The Hara ...

> And then allow the energy to drop into the soles of their feet ...

By lowering posture

> And then by powering their movements from the ground, in an ever-flowing dance

Slowly falling onto their clients

> And letting the clients totally support them whilst they work ...

Sometimes kneeling - to work in the realms of pure zero strain

> And they direct their whole body weight in order to give *shire horse* power to each movement

And in this way, Kemo-Sabe, they dance with the Dancing Bear ...

> That was fun, wasn't it, Tonto?

Most assuredly, Kemo-Sabe

🌾 🌾 🌾

> Tonto?

Yes, Kemo-Sabe?

> I feel as if I have already finished the journey!

No, Kemo-Sabe – you have only finished the hard work; now is the time to enjoy all you have achieved

> You mean the best is yet to come?

Yes, Kemo-Sabe – you do not want to miss seeing the sunrise

> Well, while we are climbing up to this Summit, Tonto, I would like to point out a few basic assumptions.

What are these, Kemo-Sabe?

> Well, firstly, this is only a book

This is true, Kemo-Sabe

> And no-one can learn bodywork from a book

So why have we spent all this time on this long journey, Kemo-Sabe? And why do we spend time describing the view and the technical details of strokes?

> Well, this is my point, Tonto. We do this merely to demonstrate how all that we have covered up to now on this journey is necessary in order fully to comprehend this new approach to massage

So this book is not a training?

No. This next bit is to show how it actually works in practice, so that our readers can see everything we have discussed in action ...

Showing how the theory we have covered is actually applied in bodywork?

Yes, Tonto. Because bodywork is an applied science ...

And an art, Kemo-Sabe; it is most assuredly first and foremost an art!

You know I agree with this, Tonto, but so much of what we have been discussing is a scientific and historical analysis of this art...

Was there anything else you wanted to say before we describe this glorious view? Quickly, see how the sun is rising!

Just one more thing, Tonto. I want to remind our fellow travellers that we are assuming that they will read this section with all their training and awareness of contra-indications in place

Kemo-Sabe, if we had taken that route and tried to describe all the contraindications to every sort of massage we have described through this land, then we would never have got to this awesome summit

So we will assume that only those who understand all the basic contraindications and necessary safeties for touch to be effective have stayed with us this far?

Yes, Kemo-Sabe, I think you can be sure of this

And look, Tonto, we have reached the Summit – at last!

Yes, Kemo-Sabe – is it not wonderful?

Yes, Tonto, it is magnificent!

So shall we describe this magnificent view, Tonto?

Most assuredly, Kemo-Sabe, most assuredly!

Tonto – tell us what you can see over to the East ...

Kemo-Sabe, I see three wondrous peaks! What about you?

I also see many peaks - let us describe them all in great detail, Tonto

Our view from the Summit?

Yes, Tonto. Our view from the Summit, the reason for this whole journey

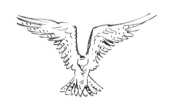

9.
THE VIEW FROM THE SUMMIT

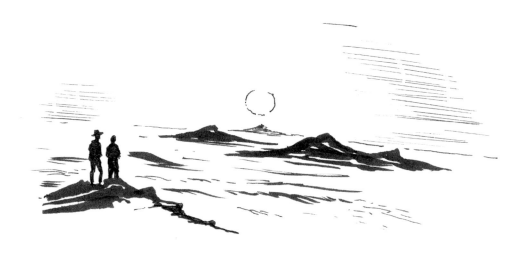

Three meridian-based Chair Massage techniques

The following meridian-based strokes are just three specific examples of how the zero-strain principles of NO HANDS Massage can be applied to the Kata taught at most seated acupressure trainings

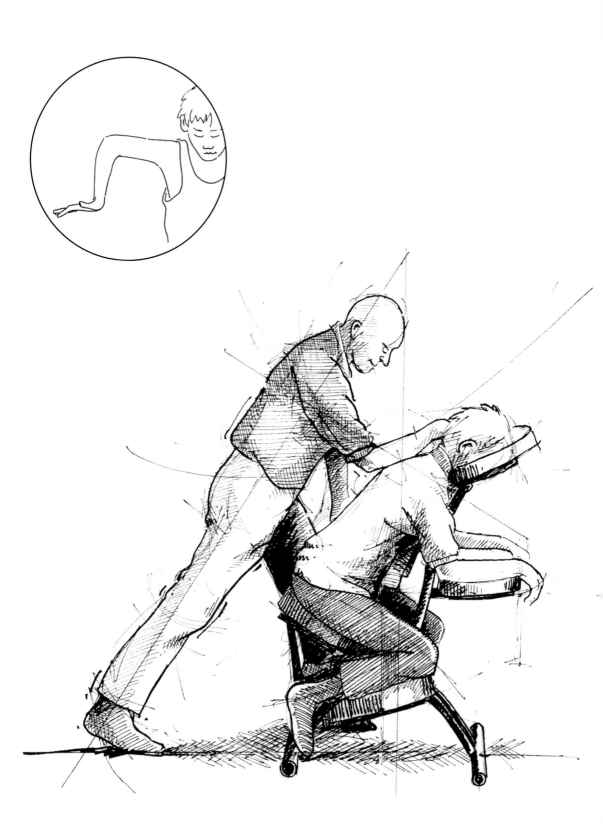

1. The Vertical Forearm Press

Main Bladder meridian between the scapula and spine

Purpose

To open up the meridian

The Vertical Forearm Press is a preparation stroke. Its function is to prepare the meridian for the point work of the elbow press which follows on immediately afterwards. It happens on the upper left and right quartiles of the body. In the sequence of the treatment Kata, it follows on from the first specific double masseur's fist.

Replacing

The Vertical Forearm Press replaces what was originally called the "archer's arm". As you can see from the smaller drawing, it is one of the most potentially damaging movements in upper body Chair Massage . The awkward angle of shoulder and elbow is not good for transferring pressure onto the client. And there are few more devastating effects on the practitioner's body than the application of large amounts of pressure onto a flexed wrist which is in contact with the relatively unyielding area of the client's back.

Description

Use the soft front of your forearm to apply gentle opening pressure to the three positions originally occupied by the "archer's arm". These are located between the spine and scapula adjacent to the superior, medial and inferior borders of the scapula. It is important to use bodyweight and to keep the forearm at 90 degrees to the client's back. As you can see from the drawing, the practitioner's bodyweight is behind and above the soft front with the back foot extended.

Practitioner contact zones used

The soft front.

Physical benefits

Practitioner: Enormous! Using the Vertical Forearm Press involves so much more than the mere avoidance of repetitive strain injury. In this position it is possible to let your whole body do the work, without having to use your arm muscles at all. When you are doing many sessions in a day this is sheer bliss and helps the Kata flow effortlessly and easily.

Client: Logically, the client should notice no difference between the two moves. In practice, however, the Vertical Forearm Press carries with it a greater sense of power than is conveyed simply by pressing the heel of the hand into the back. One is powered by arm and shoulder muscles, whilst the Vertical Forearm Press is powered by the practitioner's whole bodyweight. Clients and students who have had the benefit of both techniques report that the Vertical Forearm Press has a greater sense of nurturance than the "archer's arm". Anything that can increase this sense of nurturance for our clients, without losing effectiveness, is to be hugely welcomed. It is also true that this technique is performed a little slower than the "archer's arm", partly because of the care and attention that is given to the whole body alignment prior actually to leaning into the client's body.

Psychological benefits

This combined sense of power and nurturance is very soothing. Within the Kata so much goes on that has a psychological component! Here I believe it is all part of the opening up that goes on for a client. When I am receiving, it is a big thing to trust the practitioner to apply the correct amount of pressure and to work at a pace that suits my particular vulnerabilities at that moment. The extra nurturance, safety and postural stability that a NO HANDS approach to these movements creates, greatly helps the client at this early stage of the Kata.

Postural Considerations

The Postural Secret that is most operative in this movement is the *shire horse*. It takes a surprising amount of body-awareness to align your bodyweight securely and confidently behind this press. Ensuring that your angle of pressure is at 90 degrees to the meridian and that you are working from a stable base to avoid any wobble is surprisingly harder than first appearances!

The other Postural Secret you notice right away with this movement is *sole*. It is a concept that can radically affect the power and awareness of your work. Feeling each movement you make through both of your feet offers a new awareness of your movements. The combined effect of both these Postural Secrets is massively to increase the power of this section of the Kata.

Another Postural Secret that you notice is *falling*. This is most noticeable in the pace and depth of your transference of bodyweight into the client. Effortless it may be, but skilful it *has* to be. Even to attempt this movement on a paying client without plenty of training and experience could damage your practice and your reputation – not to mention your client's back!

As ever, the Postural Secret of Hara is present in your awareness of all your own body movements: each movement you make is more powerfully grounded and centred. These two words, grounded and centred, are bandied around in trainings, yet how often do we stop to consider what it is we actually mean by them? In Hara, I believe we have finally defined them in a precise practical and physical sense for many future generations of bodyworkers.

There is a flow to this movement, and it is a flow that fits well into our Kata. Likewise, support is experienced primarily by letting your weight fall onto the client. In particular, the triangulation principle that is a part of *support* is very noticeable here. The triangle of force runs from your feet to your shoulder and then back down to the ground through the client's body and the chair.

Safety

At the slightest sign of client discomfort or pain, the active or working arm is immediately lifted off the client. When all your weight is on the soft front, then this lift can be achieved by taking your weight fully onto your front foot and by doing an emergency back-strain lift of your torso – something normally forbidden in NO HANDS Massage but available in emergencies!

Summary

The Vertical Forearm Press is a surprisingly simple replacement of the damaging "archer's arm" technique, and it is also a powerful enhancement of the Kata. Despite its apparent simplicity, it is a movement that requires diligence be paid to all of the Postural Secrets outlined above.

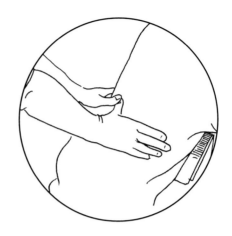

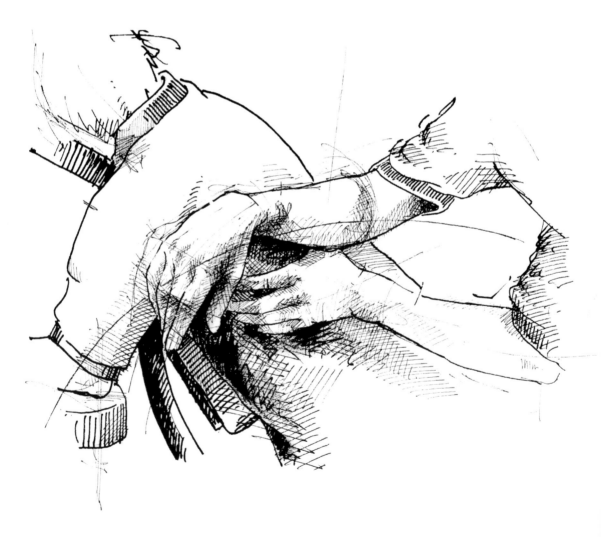

2. The Supported Thumb (lower back)

Main Bladder meridian from the inferior margin of the scapula to the iliac crest

Purpose

To apply direct pressure to the actual *tsubo* along the meridian following the more general bladder meridian work that precedes this in the Kata.

Replacing

The double thumb press. As you can see from the smaller drawing, this is usually done with one thumb on top of the other, and involves working down each side of the spine separately - from the inferior margin of the scapula down to the iliac crest. Nine *tsubo* in all are contacted on the Main Bladder meridian located on the crest of the erector spinae muscles. The lowest *tsubo* is located just above the iliac crest. Whilst this press involves less strain than the bilateral technique described below, the double thumb press still involves a lot of pressure and strain on both thumbs and wrists. For this reason, we have been searching for quite a while at the Academy for an alternative.

Some training establishments may alternatively teach this press as a bilateral technique, employing one thumb on either side of the spine simultaneously, again on the crest of erector spinae. Where this technique is used, it has to be said that practitioners have reported massive strain being placed on both the wrists and the splayed-out thumbs.

Description

With the Supported Thumb (as you can see in the drawing) a single thumb is employed (rather than one thumb on top of the other) but, in this case, the pressure is directed onto the thumb via the ulna edge of the opposite forearm. Pressure is then applied onto the back of the thumbnail through the forearm. The same nine *tsubo*, as with the replaced movement described above, are activated.

Physical benefits

Practitioner: All of the strain put onto the wrists and thumbs is eliminated by the employment of this modification. It's as simple as that! Nor is there any lack of tactile response, as the reactions of the client can be monitored just as effectively through the palmar surface of your thumb-hand. Your thumb is passive and experiences some compression, but there is absolutely no muscular activity or strain. All power and movement comes from the transfer of your bodyweight through your forearm. It is a delight to achieve all the effectiveness of this 9-point *tsubo* stimulation by simply leaning into your forearm.

Client: The flat palmar contact of your thumb-hand gives it a listening mother hand role which balances the specific *tsubo* work that is going on through the thumb. This means that the client experiences all the releases we associate with the meridian work, plus an additional nurturance from the palmar surface that is lying passively around the *tsubo* being pressed. In this sense the technique is a definite improvement on what we were using before and it is zero strain.

Postural considerations

The Postural Secret that is most operative in this movement is kneeling. This immediately eliminates any possibility of back-strain or discomfort. What has to be remembered is that the *tsubo* must be contacted through pressure that is at 90 degrees to the back. Kneeling is an effortless posture in which to achieve this angle.

As with most kneeling postures, a Postural Secret that is also active is sole. This is felt through both your feet and the knee that is acting as a foot in the proposal stance of kneeling. By feeling all your movements through your contact with the ground, you gain a stability and awareness that ensures that the *tsubo* are contacted in exactly the right manner to necessitate the flow of Ki

And this flow is the next operative Postural Secret. To move through the nine *tsubo* requires a measured flowing rhythm of forward lunging and a backward, returning movement.

Perhaps the most hidden – and possibly the most significant Postural Secret is the *shire horse*. You see, to contact the *tsubo* requires an absolute accuracy of the direction or vector of your force onto the thumb. Aligning your body behind the correct angle of pressure generally takes students a bit of time to grasp – but once you have it, then it is yours for life: zero-strain lower-back *tsubo* work.

Falling is evident in the transfer of your bodyweight through your hips into the *tsubo*. Hara is always present – in this case, it increases your own kinaesthetic awareness of your movements as well as the client's non-verbal responses to your pressure. Hara quite simply takes you deeper into your own kinaesthetic awareness and helps your bodywork to respond to feel. Support is also present as you lean into the client's back from a 90 degree angle. There is a clear triangulation running through your movements every time you contact the *tsubo.*

Safety

Because you are leaning your bodyweight through the forearm, into your thumb and onto the client's back, the safety move is immediately to release pressure by either pulling your weight back up (creating a temporary and emergency strain on your own back) or by sliding both arms off the client's body and literally falling to the floor! Sounds extreme but, if your client is in acute pain these are the safety techniques we can employ.

Summary

The Supported Thumb press replaces one of the most damaging moves that I know in Chair Massage. Not only that, it enables practitioners to get into their bodies even more – never a bad thing for a bodyworker. There is a great sense of power in this kneeling posture. Remember that it is useful to have a pillow or a cushion nearby to use as a protection for your knee!

🌿 🌿 🌿

3. Stretching – the Angel Stretch

Chest and Arm meridians

Purpose

This stretch is used when the client is returned to an upright posture at the end of the session. This is just one of a sequence of various stretches that practitioners employ to bring the client back into the real world of work and play. If the client has entered into any altered dream state during the bodywork then this work will bring them back gently into the here and now.

Replacing

This is not so much a replacement as an example of how, by simply altering our Point Of Delivery (POD), we can enter into the realms of zero strain bodywork. We normally do the Angel Stretch as part of a sequence of three stretches:

a. the Penguin or Chicken Wing stretch, followed by

b. the Angel Stretch or similar and, in some cases

c. Greet the Dawn

The Penguin stretch simply draws the elbows backwards and upwards behind the client, creating a powerful stretch to the whole upper torso. Greet the Dawn involves lifting the arms in a vertical stretch and then letting them fall down safely to the hips.

In all of these stretches we simply replace the hands with the forearms. As you can see from the smaller drawing, gripping the elbows can involve both wrist and finger strain. When we replace all of these movements with a forearm grip, we need to be very conscious of our own backs and ensure that we are not placing any damaging strain on ourselves. For the purposes of this book, we will focus simply on the Angel Stretch to demonstrate how this risk is prevented.

Description

Angel Stretch is started by asking the client to clasp their hands behind their neck and to bring their arms backwards, whilst providing support between the shoulders with your own torso. However, instead of using the palm of your hands to grip the client's forearm and make the stretch, you use your forearms to pull back the forearms – as shown in the drawing.

Whilst supporting the client's forearms in this way – and working with their breathing – bring the arms back and slightly upwards, parallel to the ground to the point of resistance. The position is taken up, the client breathes in and, as they breathe out, you make the stretch.

Your body posture consists of of bending at the knees in order to keep your own back vertical as you get your arms well underneath the client's arms. Your hips should be well tucked under your torso to provide a stable support for the upper back of the client as you make the stretch.

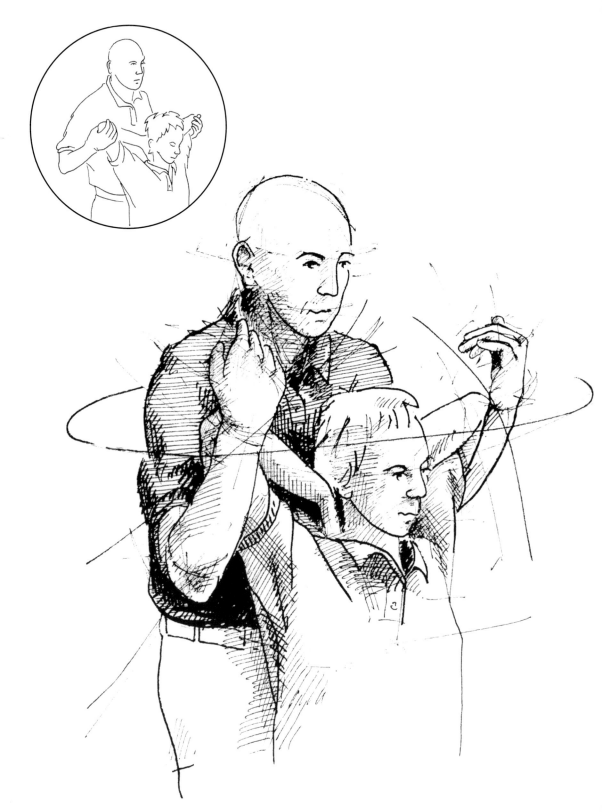

Practitioner contact zones used

The soft front.

Physical Benefits

Practitioner: Zero strain on the wrists – yet again! Gripping the elbows with your hands is a very high-strain movement. It is okay when it is done now and then – but 30 to 50 times a day? Replacing it with the forearm also brings your focus back to *yourself*: as soon as you use the forearms it is more difficult and slightly less natural to do, consequently it needs greater self-focus and body-awareness. This is something which both enhances your bodywork and protects you.

It is possible to use a great deal of power for a stretch with the forearms, something of which the client becomes aware. We never use all of this force, but the potential is clearly there. This initiates what I call the "White Flag of Surrender" from the client's tight muscles! Somatically, the client's body senses the power that you have available, and therefore it does not even bother to resist.

Client: A more nurturing effect is noticeable as more of the practitioner's forearms are in contact during the stretches. This makes the whole experience a much safer and comforting one for the client. This in turn produces a greater and more releasing stretch.

Psychological benefits

When you demonstrate enough body awareness and somatic competence to neatly "dip down" and hook the client's forearms with your own forearms, your client knows that they are in the hands of a master bodyworker! I cannot over-emphasise how important it is for your clients to have absolute trust in your physical movements and safety. NO HANDS Massage broadcasts loud and clear that you spend enormous amounts of your time and energy in the practice of all the seven Postural Secrets. This knowledge communicates itself somatically to the client. As a client, you can just feel it. You just *know*. And when you know, you let go!

Postural considerations

So the Postural Secret that is most operative in this stretch is the Hara. Opening out the client's arms to the correct amount of stretch requires a good somatic feel: it takes a great connection with your Hara to get this just right. Alongside Hara you also find that the Postural Secret of *sole* gives valuable awareness. By feeling all your movements firmly anchored in the ground you communicate solidity and security.

Bringing your whole body into each stretch involves an advanced sense of timing and flow. Your own body and the client's are locked together in a way that also activates the Postural Secret of support. The real question in this movement is "who is supporting who?" Because your torsos are locked together in the stretch, there is a fantastic mutual interdependence that is truly wonderful to experience. This is why you will always see me smiling when giving the Angel Stretch!

Safety

Any pain or discomfort is to be followed by an immediate release of the arms.

Summary

The Angel Stretch is just one example of how the forearms, as well as other body surfaces can be creatively employed to rid our profession of all injury risk – for ever. There is absolutely no need ever again to have a practitioner retire from the profession because of injury!

🌾 🌾 🌾

10.
THE VIEW
FROM THE
SUMMIT

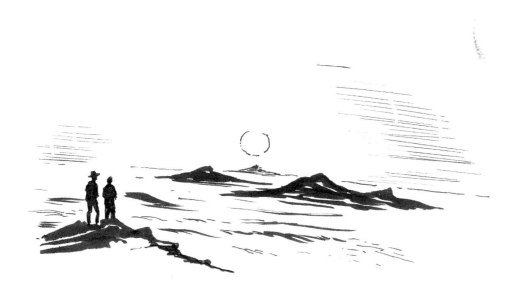

Three muscle-based
Chair Massage
techniques

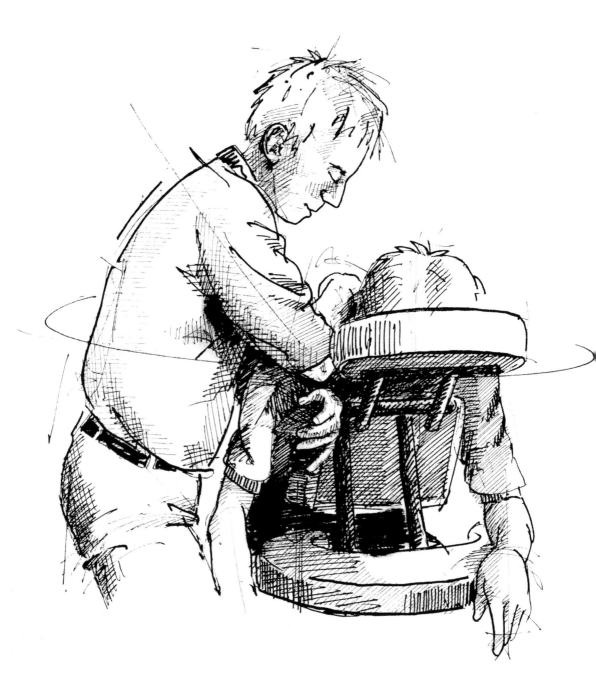

1. The Romster

Shoulder/Arm/Neck matrix

Purpose

To release the shoulder joint.

Description

Gently lift the client's arm off the arm-rest, so that it hangs down free of any contact with the chair. From a sideways-on position, you hook your arm under the client's armpit, so that you cradle the shoulder/arm/neck matrix in the crook of your arm. You then place the soft front of your other arm over the top of the client's shoulder (onto the acromium process) to make a secure 360 degrees grip.

Make sure your own back stays vertical. Rotate the client's shoulder both clockwise and anti-clockwise using your legs to power the move. This is a classic Range Of Motion (ROM) bodywork move, this is why we call it the Romster.

On the upward section of the move you are lifting the shoulder. This compresses all the muscle tissue in the matrix, and literally squashes everything towards the client's head. When you are on the downward section of the cycle, you use the soft front to press down on the shoulder and trapezius muscles. The downward movement produces a stretch for all the muscles of the matrix. This combination of "squash and stretch" makes your movements surprisingly releasing for the client. The drawing shows me at the end of the upward section of the move and just about to begin the downward section.

Pushing the whole shoulder/arm/neck matrix towards the client's head and then stretching it away from the head has a hypnotic element to it. The effortless repetition of this hypnotic move can produce powerful therapeutic effects on the client.*

Practitioner contact zones used

The soft front and the crook of your arm. One of the great things about your soft front is that it moulds so beautifully over bony protuberances like the acromium process!

Physical benefits

Practitioner: This is a powerful and dynamic move, which saves your hands from lifting the client's often very heavy shoulder girdle. Lifting the shoulder girdle is one of the most damaging movements practitioners can make with their hands but, for most ROM movements of the shoulder, the tension inherent in the hands and arms of practitioners can be removed completely. It is possible to perform this movement with so much more power and control than in conventional Western ROM movements of the shoulder and, because of the ease and comfort of this position, you can be very gentle and take as

---

*I describe this hypnotic effect in more detail on p.88 of *The Principles and Practice of NO HANDS Massage* (Pyves 2000)

long as you want to coax this area of your client's body into release and relaxation.

Client: This strong and secure grip is comforting and provides a thorough working of all the major shoulder girdle muscles. It also releases many energy blockages that can occur in this region. The gentle power of this move invites release of tension without pain. This is one of those "gentle giant" strokes – so full of potential power, yet so soft and gentle.

Psychological benefits

This grip is surprisingly comforting and facilitates the safe and relaxing release of mental and emotional tension. The client's sense of so much potential strength and power in your stance and grip, when combined with the actual gentleness of the move, is the secret to its psychological impact.

Postural considerations

For this reason, the operative Postural Secret here is the *shire horse.* By gathering your whole bodyweight behind your movements, you can effortlessly rotate and release what is a notoriously difficult zone of the body to lift and manoeuvre.

In addition to this primary Postural Secret, Hara is evident in the way this is a contained and centred movement. Once you have comfortably achieved the position, all movement seems simply to emanate from your belly. By concentrating on the Postural Secret of sole, it is possible for you to respond to the smallest shifts and releases within the client's shoulder/neck/arm matrix. This awareness enables you to make every movement powerful as well as gentle. This combination of power and gentleness is probably one of the greatest secrets behind the unbelievable effectiveness of NO HANDS Massage Flow is also key to the Romster. By working with this Postural Secret it is possible for you to lull the client into both physical and psychological release. The muscles in this area of the body are particularly susceptible to the psychological release that this flowing movement invites..

Interestingly, the Postural Secret of falling is operative, but on a very subtle level. When pushing up towards the client's head you are actually falling into the client; you are letting your bodyweight do all the work. This upward movement is powered by your legs, certainly but the real key is that, as you power up from the ground, you also *fall* into your client.

The same is true when you are pulling the shoulder/neck/arm matrix away from the head. When you do this the client is actually holding you up, and supporting you. This, then, is how the Postural Secret of support is operative.

Safety and control

At the slightest sign of client discomfort, simply release any pressure in your arms (it is essential that hard bony pressure is avoided). By keeping both arms very soft and relaxed, it is possible to get a very secure grip without causing the slightest discomfort to the client. Care must be taken not to pinch the client's skin and also to avoid the client's breast tissue.

Summary

Pareto's Principle states that 80 per cent of your results are produced by 20 per cent of your efforts – something I have found to be absolutely accurate in bodywork. I would say that the effortless repetition of the Romster can produce some of the most amazing muscular and energetic releases I have ever witnessed, and it is a stroke that bears the fruits of diligent study, training and practice. One of Pareto's 80 – 20 moves that I use every time.

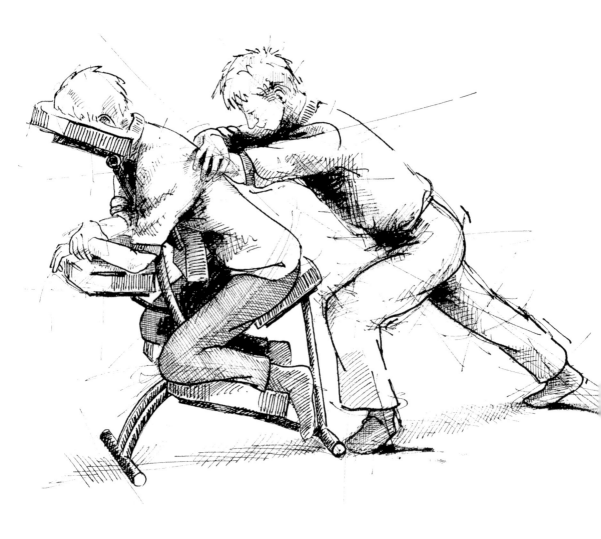

2. The Katerpillar

Erector Spinae and Sacrum

Purpose

To open up and warm the back for deeper and more muscle-specific work later on. To ease and release tension in the back (it is amazing how much tension actually disappears in the first minute of using this stroke).

Description

From a position directly posterior to the client, place the soft fronts of your forearms either side of the client's spine. To do this you have one arm above (superior to) the other. Depending on the size and shape of the client and the size and shape of your forearms, your arms may be horizontally or diagonally placed. The important thing is that only your soft fronts are applying the pressure. In this drawing my arms fit horizontally.

In this move, you are applying compressive movements. This can be done using both surfaces of your forearm either simultaneously or by alternating from one side to the other, it is called the Katerpillar, because by alternating between your arms, it is possible to walk your forearms up and down the client's spine. You can effectively work from T4 right down to the sacrum. When you reach the lower back and sacral areas, drop onto your knees. This will enable you to perform the compressive movements on this part of your client's body.

You will need some form of knee support from a cushion or thicker piece of matting for this.

Your task with the Katerpillar is to allow the client to open up and sink into the safety and expert awareness that you communicate through your touch. You will demonstrate and communicate this to your client by transferring your weight expertly.

Practitioner contact zones used

The soft front of both arms.

Physical Benefits

Practitioner: Whilst this technique begins gently and softly, it is also a powerful and dynamic move. It will 'get you into your body' and will probably 'energise' you rather than relax you. By taking a long stance, well back from the chair, you will be able to apply massive pressure without any pain to the client. By keeping one foot forward you maintain control and safety. You just focus on gentle weight transference and hold zero strain in your mind. It is possible to relax totally while you are using this technique.

Client: This technique will open up and release tension in the client's back. Like the Romster, the amount of power available to the practitioner means that some very deep muscular work can be achieved from this position. The whole back is loosened up and warmed, and a great deal of tension that sits on the top will just dissipate. It is another Pareto's Principle stroke! So much can be effortlessly achieved with this one.

Psychological benefits

At this stage, it is all about trust, . The Katerpillar is probably the first stroke you use to convey all your bodyweight into the client. With your awareness of the Postural Secrets, you convey your competency and invite the client to let go and hand over their body to you for the rest of the session. If you pass this somatic test, then the client will simply cooperate and release tension effortlessly for the rest of the session.

It is no small thing to let a person lean all their bodyweight into you. Like those wonderful trust exercises where one person catches another, it is important never to drop your client. In bodywork terms this means starting gently and increasing pressure only when, and if, the client's tissues say "yes".

Postural considerations

The operative Postural Secret here is *falling*. Central to the success of this stroke is your ability to transfer your weight from your feet to your arms. If this is done clumsily and without sufficient training, the client will just get hurt. Practising weight transference is something that should be a continual preoccupation of all NO HANDS practitioners: it must become an obsession.

In addition to *falling*, kneeling is also very active, particularly when you reach the lower back. Letting yourself slowly lunge towards the client's back from the proposal stance will power the stroke from your thighs and hips.

In this way, the Postural Secret of sole is also active, though in this case one of the soles is actually a knee. By feeling each movement you make against the floor, you are able to respond to the smallest shifts and releases within the client's muscle tissue.

Flow is also very evident in the Katerpillar - your movements are going backwards and forwards in a very flowing manner. As with all aspects of *flow*, this can help lull the client into a sense of physical and psychological release.

The Postural Secret of the *shire horse* is operative because you really do need to spend time aligning your body behind each movement. Likewise, if you Katerpillar your way down the spine, you need to create the necessary postural shifts every time you change the direction of your movements.

As you lean into the body, your client is holding you up – until your weight is transferred back into your feet. This is how the Postural Secret of support is operative.

Finally, Hara is present in this stroke as it should be in all of them. In this case it is most active in the way that you move from your feet into the client's tissues.

Safety and Control

At the slightest sign of client discomfort, simply lift your arms and drop your weight into your forward leg (if in a 'one foot forward' stance). If you have moved onto the crouch position – aka the Dancing Bear - then you drop your weight back and down into your legs. This will instantly remove all pressure from the client's back.

Summary

This is an immensely powerful stroke which, like the *shire horse,* can really plough the field of your client's tension. A great deal of the hard work can be done from this position and it is extremely pleasant to receive.

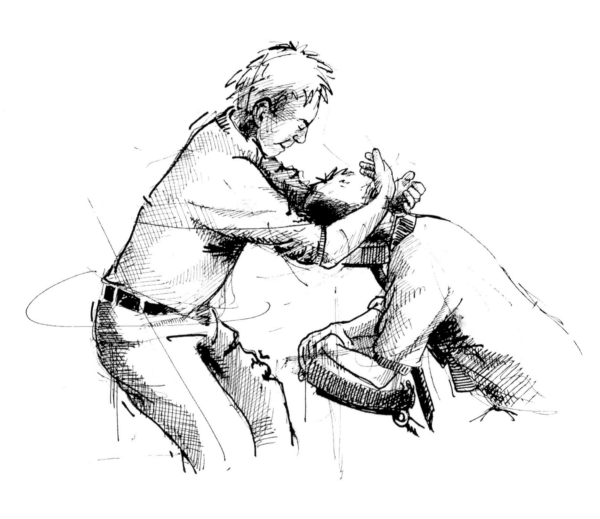

3. Dancing Tissues

Neck and Upper Back

Purpose

This stroke is used to open up and relax the muscle tissues of the upper back and neck. Doing this powerful neck work will actually give blocked energy and tension in the spine somewhere to go when it is worked on.

Description

Standing at the head of the chair, forward of the client, you place your soft fronts across the back of the client's neck. From this position you can hook onto the client's tissues at the back and side of the neck and, by moving your body create movement in the tissues, like a dance – hence the title of this technique. Much of the power in this stroke comes from the shifts you make in your body movements, turning it into a dance.

You can work both arms simultaneously or, alternatively, you can concentrate on just one side, even reaching right down the neck to the client's shoulders (trapezius muscles). The amount and depth of this work will depend on the client's receptivity and your own timing.

Practitioner contact zones used

The soft front and distal end of the ulna.

Physical benefits

Practitioner: This is a very comfortable position from which to do some very powerful neck massage. It enables you to allow your whole body movements, from the soles of your feet to the top of your head, to create the stroke. Like both the Romster and the Katerpillar, it is not so much a technique as a position from which to hook your body up with the client's body and so create the massage movements from your own body's movements.

Client: This can be a very powerful loosening of the neck and upper back muscles. It is soft, yet deep and powerful.

Psychological benefits

Perhaps the most powerful psychological aspect of this stroke is the sense of connection and togetherness that can be experienced by both practitioner and client. Togetherness: the single most significant reason for the power of all touch therapies. Here is where you can put the theory that "all massage is a dance between practitioner and client" into actual physical movements! Sometimes it is hard to put the theory into practice, but this is one of those strokes where you can really experience your massage as a dance – a dance between you and your client. It is, of course, a *pas de deux.*

Postural considerations

The operative Postural Secret here is the sole. By focusing all your awareness on the slightest changes of pressure in the soles of your feet, all your movements will be full of awareness and power. Naturally the principle of Hara is not far behind this! As you move, it is from your Hara that you make the movement. In this sense you truly can massage the client from your centre. Your arms become mere extensions of your Hara.

Nor will it surprise you to discover that flow is central to this stroke. All tissues, but particularly the neck muscles, respond well to gentle coaxing and enticement. If an animal is frightened or tense and hidden in a cave, you do not try and force it out; you get smart and entice it out with nice smells and food. So too with neck tension. Your movements must convey the sheer freedom that is possible if only they would come out and play!

Interestingly, the principle of falling is present – but in reverse. Here, the client is often supporting you as you fall backwards. You are, in effect, stopped from falling over only by your arms – which cling to your client's neck! In this way support is also active: the client is all the support you have. When you are leaning into the upper trapezius muscles, the client is also supporting you. Even when working one side of the client's neck and shoulder you will find ways to get support from the other side.

Safety and control

At the slightest sign of client discomfort you simply remove or lift your arms. Simple!

Summary

These neck muscles can hold so much tension – and very tightly! Combining a soft and gentle surface with some strong weight and pressure is an extremely effective way to invite release, all done through zero strain. This stroke is a real pleasure to give and it is possible to be lulled into believing that you could do this movement forever.

⊱─◦◦─⊰

So, Tonto, after all this travelling we get to really enjoy watching the sunset at the end of our day on top of the Summit of Chair Massage?

Most assuredly, Kemo-Sabe. We will stretch out here and soak up the glorious view

And tomorrow, Tonto?

We will walk down the other side of this Great Mountain

It looks nice and gentle, Tonto

Yes, Kemo-Sabe, it is a pleasant wooded walk

Ah, Tonto, this is the life, eh?

It most certainly is, Kemo-Sabe, it most certainly is

We can see the whole world of bodywork laid out before us – and it is so beautiful

Yes, Kemo-Sabe, you took the words right out of my mouth

Tonto?

Yes, Kemo-Sabe

Goodnight

Goodnight, Kemo-Sabe

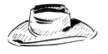

11.
WALKING DOWN THE MOUNTAIN

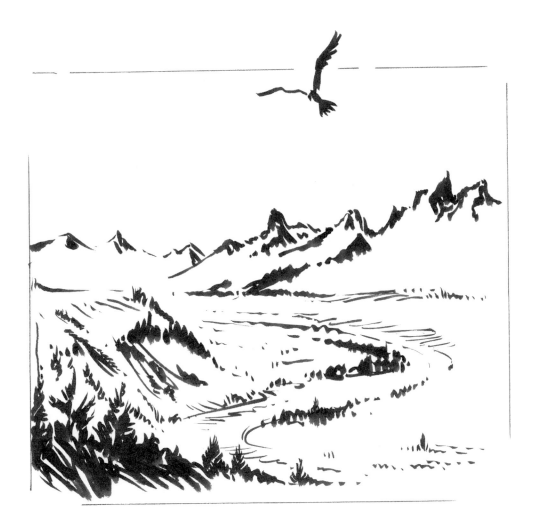

Farewell conversations

So, Tonto, this path is nice and gentle after our hard climb yesterday. Are those trees down there?

Yes, Kemo-Sabe – it is very pleasant to walk this path together in the early morning

And have we managed to demonstrate how both meridian-based and muscle-based Chair Massage can be done with zero strain?

Most assuredly, Kemo-Sabe. By putting together your revolutionary NO HANDS approach with the revolution of Chair Massage, I believe we have created the greatest bodywork revolution of them all

Well, time will tell, Tonto. The really important thing to remember, is that there is not another therapy on the planet that can provide in one session, the physical, energetic, mental and psychological healing needed by our modern world

It is hard to think of one, Kemo-Sabe.

Massage does so much more than simply realigning the structure. It detoxifies.

It connects mind to body ...

In a way, that is the envy of psychotherapists (I should know as I am one!)

It can provide the essential nurturance that is so missing in our modern-day world. This lack is the cause of who knows how many neuroses and physical symptoms, not to mention recurrent immune collapses.

It provides opportunities for the body to replenish itself after chronic depletion conditions ...

And it kick-starts the powerful self-healing mechanisms within the body.

And bodyworkers are daily addressing and soothing and releasing the massive psychological tension of our stressful and environmentally compromised modern lives, Tonto

Yes, Kemo-Sabe, they do this through the phenomenal power of soothing touch, so that none of the weird and wonderful syptomatology that the human body is capable of ever emerges in the first place

And in many cases, Tonto, massage therapists are soothing the transition from this world to the next in hospices right across the world.....

Like the shaman, Kemo-Sabe

Yes, Tonto.

🌿 🌿 🌿

Kemo-Sabe?

> What is it, Tonto?

All this is wonderful. But how is it that so many practitioners seem to struggle to build up practices?

> Well, it's important to point out that massage practitioners are trying hard to survive in a culture where people do not yet know enough about the wonderful benefits of touch

Which is why Chair Massage is so terribly important, Kemo-Sabe

> Yes, Tonto. Otherwise how will the public learn about touch? We need to open our eyes to the cultural, political and social contexts in which we are working; we need to become ambassadors of touch in order to have an impact on the world. There is only one group of people who can do this – us! It's no good sitting around waiting for someone else to do this for us

So getting out there to display and advertise our work through Chair Massage is one of the many ways that massage practitioners and massage as a profession can show the world the power of touch

> Yes, Tonto. And whenever one bodyworker passes another in the street who does Chair Massage they should shake hands and thank them for promoting the profession ...

And then get on the chair and pay them for a session just to support them!

> Yes, Tonto, even bodyworkers who know how powerful touch is don't always book enough sessions for themselves. And if all the bodyworkers in the planet paid for weekly massage, then there would be no such thing as a practitioner without clients!

And how can they expect the public, who do not always know about these benefits, to book regular sessions for themselves?

> Exactly! Two things would happen if bodyworkers booked regular sessions for themselves ...

Well, firstly, that's a lot of well-massaged practitioners, Kemo-Sabe!

> Yes, and secondly, how much more impressive as ambassadors of touch will these well-massaged practitioners be to the public?

They will be glowing with the radiance of health, Kemo-Sabe!

> And people will be asking them what their secret is, so they do not even have to try to market themselves; their health will do it for them

That is three things, Kemo-Sabe

> So it is

I like the sound of this lazy form of marketing Kemo-Sabe!

> Yes, so do I. And look, I can see the end of the path – we are almost at the base of the Mountain!

Kemo-Sabe?

Yes, Tonto?

What happens now?

I think it is time to move on, Tonto

Where will you go now, Kemo-Sabe?

Well, Tonto, there is a land called Reflexology that has been calling strongly to me these last two years

NO HANDS Reflexology, Kemo-Sabe?

Yes, Tonto

That sounds like a good place to go, Kemo-Sabe

Yes, Tonto. Many fine bodyworkers are being injured in that land and I would like to help out as much as I can

That is good, Kemo-Sabe

Yes, Tonto, it is

🌿 🌿 🌿

Kemo-Sabe?

Yes, Tonto?

I cannot guide you through this land of Reflexology,

I know, Tonto, I know

Who will look after you in this land, Kemo-Sabe?

I will find a good scout and guide, Tonto

Oh

🌿 🌿 🌿

Kemo-Sabe?

Yes, Tonto?

Will you make sure this guide can take you safely across this land of Reflexology, Kemo-Sabe?

Yes, I will find a great master and teacher like you

Then that is good, Kemo-Sabe

Yes, Tonto, it is.

🌿 🌿 🌿

Kemo-Sabe?

Yes, Tonto?

We have reached the base of the Mountain now

I know, Tonto, I know

And my way lies back east in this direction ...

And mine in another ...

I am sad, Kemo-Sabe

Me too, Tonto

🌿 🌿 🌿

So it is time to say goodbye, Kemo-Sabe?

Yes, it is

I liked the Dancing Bear, bit, Kemo-Sabe!

Me too, Tonto, me too

What a magnificent creature he is!

The very best, Tonto

🌿 🌿 🌿

Kemo-Sabe?

Yes, Tonto?

The journey was good, wasn't it ?

Yes, it was good, Tonto!. It was worth every minute and I will never forget it – and you have plenty in your saddlebag to remind you of all that we have learned.

Thank you for being such good company and such a wise scout, Tonto

Thank you for taking me with you, Kemo-Sabe

It has been a privilege. Goodbye Tonto

Farewell, Kemo-Sabe!

🌿 🌿 🌿

The End

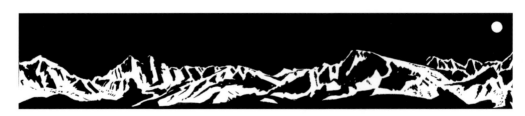

APPENDIX

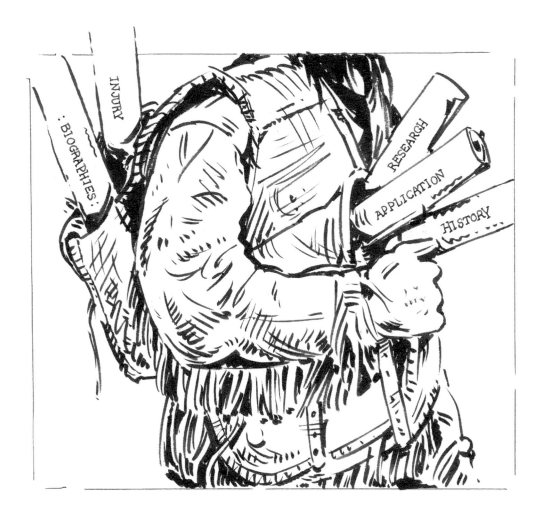

Tonto's saddlebag:

a. Biographies

The Lone Ranger's Story

So the pain shot through my arm like hot, burning, liquid metal ...

My own tale of massage injury is told in my book *NO HANDS Massage-Zero Strain Bodywork*. In it I describe how I became injured through the use of techniques that I had been taught by my excellent and gifted teachers. In it I describe my journey of discovery into my own healing and into the massage profession's 'injury secret'.

Since that book I have been going around conferences and exhibitions to the sound of loud support and cheering, telling my story, blowing the whistle on our industry's neglect of this most important issue and showing how my zero-strain approach can uphold the finest and most ancient bodywork traditions in the world.

Several hundred trained practitioners later, I have been privileged to witness so many massage careers being saved that I wake up every day with a smile - simply knowing that today there is going to be healing touch going on out there that would not have happened. Because those practitioners had already given up! And that I am responsible for the birth of a massively growing army of practitioners who will never, ever get injured!

And I smile at my dream of an association of octogenarian practitioners who dance and giggle their way through the agenda of their raucous meetings, throwing custard tarts at anyone who takes themselves too seriously. And that conference room is brim-full of truly healthy masters of the healing arts of touch who daily 'bring through' and help the newcomers in our profession.

"Soon, soon", I say to myself.

And I smile at how the words and touch of my first massage trainer completely messed my life up! Prior to this I had only had a passing interest in massage. After the transformational experiences of this training I was, quite simply, an addict of touch. Out of the window went a promising career as a history teacher, out of the window went any job security or pension plan. And in came excitement, fulfilment and meaning. It was a good trade.

And meanwhile, after the publication of my first book, practitioner after practitioner asked me, "When can you bring out the Chair Massage book?". For several years I had been noticing how, despite the best efforts of the greatest teachers in Chair Massage the thumbs were getting it in the neck, so to speak!

And still I waited ...

Practitioners really don't believe me when I say it took me twenty years to develop this simple No Hands approach outlined in my first book ...

Yet it's true.

Just as in a bodywork session, timing is the key – how there is a moment when it is right just to be still, and there is a moment when it is imperative to work like a whirling dervish and hold nothing back!

So timing is the key in everything - timing is "it" in bodywork! And the same is true with writing. So after my NO HANDS Massage book came out, I waited ... learning, watching, all the while receiving bodywork from Chair Massage practitioners. Waiting ...

Waiting for what?

I didn't know it at the time, but I was waiting for a true master of Chair Massage to arrive and build this book with me ...

And then one day, he arrived – in the foyer of a Rochdale Travel Inn!

"Hello " he said with a smile in his eyes that had "mischief" and "scallywag" written right across it!

"My name's David Woodhouse". And he offered a handshake that would have warmed the cockles of your heart …

"Shall we do some bodywork?" - part challenge part playfulness!

"I hear you can do a thing or two with your hands – or without them, eh?." That twinkle in his eye again!

And sitting on the Chair as his touch melted my muscles and attended to my tensions

I knew absolutely and immediately

That here was the one I had been waiting for …

A Tonto for this very lonely Lone Ranger!

And then, as I worked on his body and felt his tissues dance and respond with ripples of laughter and release I knew for certain, that

This team could really travel far together!

🌿 🌿 🌿

Tonto's Story

My own background had absolutely nothing to do with bodywork.

Being born in the City of Stoke-on-Trent, England, I had followed several generations of my family into the pottery industry and spent a few years learning all about the intricacies of design – the difference between china and earthenware and so on, but all from the sales side.

After some eighteen years with one company and having reached the dizzy heights of main board director, I was to find out in 1991 that the first people to go in the event of a company crash were the sales team!

The following three years were pretty amazing.

As I tried to find job security again, I decided to turn an interest in massage into something more tangible, so I enrolled on a two-year therapeutic and remedial massage course in Bristol. Great foundation training! As I was a fair way into that, I 'found' On-Site Massage quite by accident and, to cut a long story short, went down to Brighton to train in that special something which began to change my life. Chair Massage... Wow!

I reckon that after the first weekend's training I must have driven home about 6 feet above the road, I was so bowled over by the whole concept.

What is it about the power of touch that makes us stop, and look and listen anew?

I felt as if that 'fickle finger of fate' had suddenly pointed down at me and said: "'Bout time you looked at your life old son. There's something better for you out there.'

So 1991 started that old roller coaster when my head was turned inexorably and inevitably towards this wonderful profession of ours and names, events, dates, locations - all combined to mould the life of a guy who had had nothing more than a platonic interest in touch into something more exciting, vibrant and downright earth-shattering.

Gone was the thirty-year association with the ceramics industry …

Gone was working in the corporate world with its inevitable 'dark suit' image, interminable meetings and ladder-climbing.

In came the sheer challenge (and fright!) of self-employment.

In came the knowledge that there would never again be the comfort zone of a salary cheque at the end of each month.

In came an association and friendship with some of the most talented, sincere and downright wonderful people that I have ever had the good fortune to meet.

Like Gerry, I have given many talks over the years to a great number of people, both within our profession and away from it, and I am often left smiling at the way in which my life-journey took such a U-turn. I marvel at each turn and twist:

- wondering if massage had a broader connotation that its erstwhile red light image
- finding a training school reasonably locally with spaces on its two-year course
- marvelling at the power of touch and its profound effects on both the giver and the receiver
- struggling with A and P homework!
- cursing the person who had cancelled an appointment one fateful Wednesday evening
- reading a magazine with an article on 'On Site' seated acupressure massage whilst waiting for my next client
- joining the very next course
- falling in love with a therapy which had touched me deeper than anything ever had before
- joining the tutor ranks
- being offered the opportunity to buy the Academy of On Site Massage
- seeing The Academy grow with the help of some inspirational colleagues
- expanding into the realms of equipment supply with the opening of two massage-table stores
- meeting Gerry in the foyer of a Travel Inn and exchanging remarkable bodywork with this gifted maverick!

And I was delighted to discover that Gerry and I shared the same passion for our chosen pathway through life: a desire to spread the word of something quite unique and to share that passion with anyone who chooses to listen.

And I was to have the privilege of working with some of the most dedicated and talented people on this planet

Travel? Why not?

Saddle up, Lone Ranger. I'm right there with you!

b. Injury

Injurious Massage Techniques – A Silence of the lambs?

This is the first of three articles written by Gerry Pyves and published in Today's Therapist *regarding the massage profession's use of damaging techniques. This first article addresses the issue of musculo-skeletal damage that practitioners may be causing themselves through conventional techniques. In the second article Gerry Pyves examines the historical reasons for our emphasis on these injury-producing techniques. In the third article he writes about his own zero-strain approach to bodywork and massage.*

Recent research and literature in the field of massage and bodywork has opened up the debate on the way in which practitioners are using their bodies. This article summarises developments that are relevant to any practitioner who uses their hands.

A study in the UK has discovered that out of 266 massage, and aromatherapy practitioners, 207 had experienced injury of some kind or another that could be related directly to their bodywork. This represents a staggering 78 per cent (Watson 2000). This research was undertaken to assess the actual extent of injury experienced by massage professionals, following anecdotal evidence, of injury suffered by bodyworkers in America, in a book for massage practitioners entitled "Save Your Hands" by Lauriann Greene (1995). Greene, who started studying massage in America, soon found that the techniques she was taught were causing her debilitating pain and injury. Greene's frustration and annoyance led her to examine in more depth what it was that she was being expected to do by her teachers.

In conjunction with her brother, Dr. Robert Greene, a clinical assistant professor of medicine, she made some alarming discoveries. She found that the type of repetitive movements being asked of massage students fitted into the high-risk category of injury-producing movements. She writes:

> *"Except for those massage therapists who do mostly very light techniques (e.g. energy balancing or craniosacral work), most practitioners will experience some kind of injury or pain syndrome at some point in their careers as a result of giving massages."(Greene 1995)*

This led her to re-evaluate her approach and to look at the profession from the practitioner's point of view. She ran workshops on injury prevention and found that practitioners began to talk about injuries they had developed since practising massage. Perhaps one of Greene's greatest contributions was to open up the debate on professional injury, and make it acceptable for practitioners to talk about their injuries. Prior to this there had been a 'silence of the lambs', most probably explained by the shame that practitioners may have felt in having to admit that they had hurt themselves. Greene now has a regular column in one of the American massage magazines, in which practitioners write about health problems they experience due to using massage techniques. Unfortunately Greene was injured during her training and was unable to practise as a therapist:

> *"Since I could no longer give hands on massages I decided to use my training to research and write about occupation-related upper extremity injury" (1995, p.4)*

Her lack of clinical experience as a practitioner, however, made it impossible for her to identify more than partial solutions to the problems she wrote about. What practitioners require is a totally effective technical solution to what appears to be an "injury pandemic".

In the UK, another massage student, Alison Adams, presented a paper as part of her training in which she coined the phrase "Masseurs Degenerative Syndrome". In this she examined the stages of injury common to all over-use injuries, and related this to massage techniques. Adams, a nurse tutor, discovered that when we study in detail the process of injury to bones, ligaments, tendon and muscle we find that abnormal loading creates micro-injury, which can then lead to serious long-term chronic injury. Both Adams and Greene concur in considering massage to be an activity that creates considerable 'abnormal loading' to the practitioners fingers and wrists. Whilst Greene maintained that practitioner awareness would help solve the problem (1995, p.16), Adams identified that this is not the case – there are in fact seven stages of massage-injury as a direct result of abnormal loading; the figure is based on existing medical literature.

The Seven Stages of Injury

Stage 1: Abnormal Pressure

This can be created by repeating even very light movements many times during a day

As the tissues become fatigued even normal loading can begin to cause strain

Stage 2: Fatigue

Abnormal pressure results in tissue exhaustion and loss of elasticity, creating the brittleness necessary for damage

This in turn results in normal loading being experienced as abnormal loading by tissues

Stage 3: Repeated Micro-Trauma

The first damage occurs in the form of micro-stress fractures to the bones as well as micro-ruptures to tendons and muscles

Normal loading now experienced as abnormal and even painful (eg. lifting saucepan and turning handles become painful)

As tissues become deformed, the resulting inefficiency of tissues and joints creates additional fatigue and micro-trauma

Stage 7: Disability

This is when retirement or career-change is no longer an option, but enforced, with all the financial, social and emotional damage that this entails

Stage 6: Resultant Medical Conditions

Untreated and unrested, the situation becomes sufficiently painful for the sufferer to need to seek medical advice and the following conditions are identified:

oseoporosis, osteoarthritis, tendonitis, carpal tunnel syndrome, repetitive strain injury, inflammatory arthritis, nerve impingement injury, overuse syndrome

Stage 5: Delayed Long-Term Injury

It is only at this stage that the practitioner experiences more than the occasional twinge during massage. Pain continues after exertion. By this time the damage cannot be repaired quickly through the body's normal healing responses. The severity of the injuries at this stage means that the body needs months of rest to repair itself

Stage 4: Micro-Deformation

These repeated traumas stimulate abnormal bone growth and scar tissue

Key point:

The practitioner only experiences serious pain at Stage 5, occasional twinges at Stage 4, and no pain before this

Perhaps Adams most shocking discovery was that the practitioner only begins to notice injury at the fourth stage, when the injury itself is already serious and the damage is on the verge of becoming permanent. This means that no matter how self-aware the practitioner is, abnormal loading causes injuries that are well established before any aches and pains are experienced by the practitioner. Micro-traumas to muscle tissue and joint capsules and micro-fractures to bones may have already occurred by the time any physical symptoms are experienced. This means that, for the practitioner, the slightest ache could be merely the tip of an injury iceberg. Refusal to make changes or to rest can lead to permanent damage.

In the study undertaken by Watson (2000) to assess the actual scope of the problem that Greene and Adams had identified, massage practitioners were asked to identify any injuries to their hands or wrists that had developed, subsequent to learning and practising massage. They were also asked about any deterioration of previous injuries. This information was collated, alongside information about the numbers of massage treatments that practitioners were giving, into a report entitled: "An investigation into the links between massage practice and musculo-skeletal damage to the practitioner's hands and wrists" . The results show that 78 per cent of respondents to the study have experienced injury. What is perhaps the most worrying is that these statistics only represent practitioners who have already reached the fourth stage of injury or beyond and are aware of the damage that has been caused to their tissues. Given that this fourth stage is half-way through the injury process, this could easily mean that similar numbers of practitioners are also undergoing the first three stages of injury. As a result, a more accurate figure for practitioner damage could be well over 90 per cent.

How is it possible that massage practitioners are using techniques that are so damaging?

In my next article "Massage History – From Technique to Therapy"(Pyves G. 2000c), I argue that the massage techniques taught by Per Henrik Ling (1776-1839) who is generally regarded as the father of Western massage, were never intended to be used in the intensive way that they are now used. Ling himself only used massage as an adjunct to exercise and stretching in his 'Swedish Movement Cure'. Nowadays, practitioners are using the same massage techniques consistently and exclusively for up to 50-90 minutes at a time. I also argue that massage as a therapeutic discipline has adapted itself to the needs of stressful modern society and has transformed itself into a therapy in its own right. In other words massage is now used in an entirely different way and in a totally different setting than in Ling's day.

Another reason for the continuing use of damaging techniques may be the 'alternative' and independent culture of much massage therapy. This has meant that, until recently, massage therapy has avoided the rigorous attention of employment legislation. As massage becomes more mainstream, it is likely that we will see a lot of attention being focused on what constitutes healthy practise in the work place by both unions, professional associations and employers. Nurses underwent such scrutiny in the 1960s in the UK that resulted in nurses being forbidden to lift patients unless a winch was available. What massage techniques will survive such scrutiny?

Significantly, Greene (1995) has pointed out that the pressure exerted on massage therapists by insurance companies in the USA has added to the likelihood of strain and injury. As many of these insurance-funded sessions are to do with structural problems, practitioners often resort to high-pressure digital techniques that are the most damaging.

'Health and Safety at Work' legislation makes employers now legally liable for any injury sustained by their employees whilst at work. As a result of this, much attention has been focused on occupational injuries such as RSI and carpel tunnel injuries for office workers. New keyboard and seating technologies have been developed, as well as trainings in posture at work for office workers. It seems ironic that so much attention has been focused on office work when, for office workers to get anywhere near the amount of strain that massage practitioners daily place on their fingers and wrists, they would have to put their whole bodyweight behind each tap of the keyboard.

Does this mean we should abandon massage? Should we abandon any hope for totally healthy massage practitioners?

Archaeological findings suggest that humans were happily massaging ointments into each other over 50,000 years ago. Over the last two centuries we have accrued much evidence of the medical benefits of massage. The current renaissance in massage is producing a plethora of research into the physical, mental and emotional benefits of massage, most especially through the work of Dr Tiffany Field at the Touch Research Institute, Miami. We know there is nothing wrong with the effects of massage; what practitioners need are new methods for applying the strokes; we need to discover, in the light of this new evidence of practitioner damage, what techniques we can use that cause zero –strain to practitioners.

It is my contention that it is simply not possible to perform massage using traditional strokes without practitioners damaging their hands. No matter how healthy the practitioner, or how careful the practitioner, these strokes are intrinsically damaging. We can keep walking around this problem or we can solve it. Carrying on trying to find harmless ways of applying harmful traditional strokes is attempting to "square the circle". It is necessary for the profession as a whole to solve this problem with a total solution. NO HANDS Massage is a practitioner solution that totally solves the problem of practitioner damage. It is for bodyworkers who want to build successful practices.

In my own clinical work, due to injury to my own wrists, I have spent the last ten years developing zero-strain techniques. I write about this new advanced bodywork technology in my book *NO-HANDS Massage* (Pyves, 2000a) which has been written and published to address the issue of practitioner damage. I believe the solution lies in abandoning the hands completely for almost all our bodywork and utilising the many other appropriate surfaces of our body that are available. For this practitioners must see themselves as "dancers" and be experts in their own movement awareness.

My new bodywork technology (requiring a technical rethink on every aspect of the practitioner's own movements) encourages practitioners to see every bodywork session as a Tai Chi meditation or a yoga session – for themselves. It identifies the value and encourages the practice of a healing synergy in which both practitioner and client experience the benefits of giving and receiving healing touch. It is no longer acceptable to focus purely on the benefits for the client. The traditional paradigm of the healer "giving" healing to the client is simply inaccurate for bodywork. Most bodyworkers are in bodywork because of the self-healing that is triggered by giving massage and we do not need to be ashamed of this. Massage practitioners must now ask themselves, "How does this technique benefit me?" A sick and injured practitioner is no use to anyone; a healthy and vibrant practitioner can help heal a touch-starved society.

Information regarding the new form of bodywork NO HANDS Massage can be obtained by contacting The NO HANDS Massage Co. on 0870 2430876 or by visiting the website: www.nohandsmassage.com

This article was first published by Shi'Zen Publications Summer 2000.

References:

Adams, A. "Degenerative Masseurs Syndrome" Workshop presentation 2000

Benjamin, P.J. "The Seeds of a Profession" The Massage Journal 41-47 1988

Cassar, M.P. *The Massage Handbook* 1999

Downing, G. *The Massage Book* 1972

Greene, L. *Save Your Hands* 1995

Greene, L. "How to become a massage athlete" Massage Magazine May/June 1999

Mackereth, P. (Lecturer in complementary studies, Salford University) - personal communication

Mills S. and Budd, S. "Professional Organisation of Complementary and Alternative medicine in the UK 2000" A second report to the Dept of Health. University of Exeter. 2000

Porter Dr R. 2000 (Professor of History of Medicine, Wellcome Trust, UK) - Personal communication

Pyves G. *NO-HANDS MASSAGE – A revolution in Bodywork* Shi'Zen Publications 2000a.

Pyves G. *Massage Techniques are damaging Practitioners Hands* Shi'Zen Publications 2000b

Pyves G. *Massage History – From Technique to Therapy* Shi'Zen Publications 2000c

Pyves G. *NO-HANDS MASSAGE – A New Bodywork Technology* Shi'Zen Publications 2000d.

Tappan F. Healing Massage Techniques, Holistic, Classic and Emerging Methods" 1980 Appleton and Lange

Tracey C. "Massage Then and Now" Massage Winter 1992/3

Watson D. *An investigation into the links between massage practice and musculo-skel;etal damage to the practitioner's hands and wrists* Shi'Zen publications 2000

Van Der Why R.P. "Of What Value is the Swedish Movement Cure?" Massage Therapy Journal Winter 1993)

Van der Why R.P. Personal communication, 2000

═➤〇◄═

c. Massage History from technique to therapy

This is the second in a series of three articles published in Today's Therapist *in which I address the issues of the historical roots of massage and its evolution as a therapy*

Personal interest

My interest in the history of massage stems from my experience of being a massage practitioner over the last fifteen years. In the first few years, I damaged my wrists whilst building a busy and successful practice and this forced me to explore different ways of providing my clients with the beneficial effects of massage without damaging myself. Over ten years of intensive clinical experimentation and workshop presentations, I created a new system of massage that totally abandoned the use of hands for any work requiring pressure. I write about this in my book *NO HANDS Massage* (Pyves 2000a).

Let me say at once that good bodywork does not require pressure. Some of the most powerful effects of massage stem from the analgesic and reflex effects of light touch. These benefits are the result of what I term 'systemic massage'. Massage has an impact on all the body systems, through the stimulation of the nervous system, and amongst others, the changes made to the client's muscle and connective tissue 'sheath'. This 'systemic massage' can be achieved with or without deep pressure. Such benefits are achieved through sustained and continuous massage for up to fifty minutes. These repetitive movements can be as damaging to the hands as high-intensity structural 'problem-solving' techniques (Pyves, 2000b, Greene 1995). Whatever style of bodywork is needed, NO HANDS Massage provides a total clinical and technical solution to the problem of practitioner damage.

Practitioner injury

Recently, there has been an upsurge of interest in practitioner damage that confirmed my own experiences (Greene 1995, Adams 2000). A report into massage work in the UK showed that up to 78 per cent of full time bodyworkers were experiencing pain and injury to wrists and fingers that indicated the presence of damaged tissues (Watson 2000). Given that massage is largely a self-employed and unregulated profession, and that by the time an injury is noticed the practitioner is already at the fourth of seven stages of injury (see Adams 2000) this could be just the tip of an injury iceberg.

Consequently, I found myself asking the question, "Why are massage practitioners now experiencing injury to their wrists and fingers through techniques that we know have been used successfully for centuries?" To answer this I needed to look at how the practice of Western massage has changed over the last 200 years.

Massage roots

Traditions of massage can be found dating as far back as the beginning of written records. Prehistoric artefacts suggest even earlier beginnings to this most natural of healing arts. The 'father' of Western massage, however, is generally regarded to be Per Henrik Ling (1776-1839) who developed the 'Swedish Movement Cure'. In 1939 the American Medical Association celebrated Ling on the centenary of his death as "The father of physical therapy" (Van der Why, 1993). In Ling's 'Movement Cure', massage techniques were used as part of a programme of movement, exercise and stretching, based on the newly discovered knowledge of the circulation of the blood and lymph. In this, Ling contributed greatly to the development of a new science called "Gymnastics".

He himself may have been influenced by the earlier reputation and writings of Francis Fuller in England and Joseph-Clement Pissot in France, both of whom used massage as part of their pioneering work in exercise and movement (Cassar, 1999). There may have been other influences, but it is beyond the scope of this article to examine the origination of Ling's techniques.

The Swedish Cure

The massage component was not particularly emphasised in Ling's 'Movement Cure'. It was only much later that this aspect of his work was taken out of context and became known as "Swedish Massage". Ling himself was fascinated by the way in which habitual restricted movements interfered with health. He was one of the first people to teach bodily movements systematically. In this he was the precursor many traditions of movement and exercise therapy, perhaps most notably of F. M. Alexander's (1865-1955) 'technique' and the "Awareness through Movement" approach of Moshe Feldenkreis (1904–1984) . Ling was never interested in massage strokes being used on their own; his Movement Cure consisted of different movements that were classified according to who performed them. These were:

1 *Active movements*: these were strengthening, stretching and mobilisation exercises performed by the client.

2 *Duplicated movements*: these involved the combined work of client and practitioner, both assistive and resistive. This involved, typically, stretches and resisted movements.

3 *Passive movements*: these involved movements performed by the practitioner or 'gymnast'. Typically these involved joint mobilisations, passive stretches and massage strokes.

Thus we can see that Ling's system was an ordered system involving exercises, stretches, resisted movements, a range of motion exercises, passive stretches, and massage strokes. Ling trained physicians to make assessments and to make a prescription in shorthand for lay practitioners to apply. These lay practitioners (gymnasts) would then carry out the movement cure (Van der Why, 1993). Of all the techniques they were asked to carry out, massage strokes applied by the 'gymnast' formed less than one sixth of the treatment. For this reason, many of the early drawings of Ling's work show mobilisation and Range of Motion diagrams, as much as massage strokes.

Ling was not trained in medicine and often used poetic and mystical language in his writings. This possibly hindered his acceptance by the Swedish medical community. Eventually, however, with the support of his influential clients, Ling established the Royal Gymnastic Central Institute in Stockholm in 1813. It is from this establishment that many of the historical roots of Western massage spring. Ling trained many physicians who then spread his ideas worldwide. One of these, M LeRon, brought the Movement Cure to Russia, and established a clinic in St Petersburg. Another, the English physician Mathias Roth (also a pioneer in the homeopathic movement) brought 'the Cure' to England and wrote the first book about Ling's work. Two of Roth's own students, Charles Fayette Taylor and George Henry Taylor brought the Swedish Movement Cure to America in 1856. In all of these countries very strong traditions of Ling's Movement Cure have subsequently evolved.

Massage was still mainly a Movement Cure even by the end of the nineteenth century. The compilers of the 1911 Encyclopaedia Britannia describe 'massage' as:

> *Where the operator moves the limbs while the patient resists, thus bringing the opposing muscles into play.*

Earlier on in this article I mentioned the value of light touch. In this context, the link between early massage and homeopathy is interesting. Many of the pioneers of early massage, published their articles about the benefits of the Movement Cure in national homeopathic journals. In 1856, for example, Mathias Roth published an article in the British Journal of Homeopathy entitled "On the prevention of illness through movements". In America, his student, George Henry Taylor did likewise. The homeopathic principle of "treat like with like" was translated into treating a movement disorder with more movement. Likewise the homeopathic principle of "Infinitesimals" suggested that the more dilute the dose, the more powerful the remedy. When this was translated into bodywork, Roth suggested there was a strong argument for emphasising the use of light techniques (Van der Why 2000). It is interesting that the many powerful modern bodywork systems that still emphasise the beneficial effects of light touch continue these homeopathic principles.

Swedish massage strokes

In modern parlance, Ling's original system was a health enhancement programme that used massage alongside exercise and stretching to promote hygiene and prevent illness. This is the context in which the five major 'Swedish Massage' techniques of Effleurage, Petrissage, Tapotement, Friction, and Vibration were developed. Ling himself did not use these names. The first use of these now familiar terms was by followers of an influential Dutch physician, Dr Johanne Mezger (1839-1909). Mezger was influential in bringing massage to the scientific community of his day (Benjamin 1980).

It has perplexed many massage tutors and students why these French words have been universally used to describe these five core massages techniques, some suggesting that the techniques themselves originated in France. As the early history of massage encompasses so much more than merely French history, it led me to look into the practices of this period. I was not surprised to discover that Mezgar's use of French is entirely consistent with the use of this language by the international medical and scientific community of the day (Porter R. 2000). It was because Mezger was so keen to promote the benefits of massage to the medical community of his day that he used French words for these techniques. Physicians throughout the nineteenth century were fascinated by the benefits of massage and much valuable research was done on it during this time. This is the most probable explanation for the now universal use of these French terms.

These five core techniques became the foundation of almost every massage and bodywork training throughout the world. What is significant is that Ling himself only used them as part of an integrated system of exercise, stretching and movement therapy. This means that massage was never used by Ling as a therapy in its own right, but more as an adjunct to his Movement Cure. The massage techniques were therefore only used for short amounts of time.

The nineteenth century

Many later medical uses of massage followed this piecemeal use of massage techniques. It seems that massage techniques were used in a variety of settings to treat specific complaints. Charles Tracey, in his article "Massage, Then and Now" (1992/3), writes of the nineteenth century:

Massage at this period was seen strictly as an adjunct to medical treatment, rather than a form of relaxation, and it was very often used in association with electrotherapy.

Of the duration of sessions, he also says:

Massage sessions tended to be much shorter than today. This must have been because they were conducted by the physician himself and would tend to concentrate on a limited medical problem.

Research is emerging that supports the idea that massage in these medical settings was performed fairly rapidly for only short periods of time (Mackereth, P, 2000). In the nineteenth century then, following in Ling's footsteps, massage was primarily a collection of techniques to be used as an adjunct to another therapy. It was most definitely not a therapy in its own right.

It is interesting to note that even when used in such intermittent ways, these techniques presented problems of strain to practitioners. That these techniques are intrinsically damaging was acknowledged by both George Henry Taylor and Sondar in the late 1850's in America by their simultaneous creation of machines to duplicate the effects of massage strokes. The reason given by Taylor was that they were proving "debilitating to the practitioner". (Van der Why 2000)

The twentieth century

In the twentieth century and especially since the early 1960s, massage and bodywork have experienced a massive transformation both in their resurgent popularity and in the way they are applied. Massage has transformed itself into a therapy in its own right, with sessions often lasting for an hour or more, consisting almost exclusively of the application of massage strokes. During this time we also saw the birth of a plethora of creative and powerful bodywork therapies many of which trace their roots back to 'Swedish Massage'. The following list is an example of some of these.

Bodywork Therapies

Alexander Technique, Bioenergetics, Heller Work, Osteopathy, Therapeutic Touch, Anthroposophical Medicine, Bowen Techniques, Mechanotherapy, Pfrimmer Technique, Touch for Health, Aromatherapy, Chiropractic, Muscle Energy Technique, Polarity Therapy, Tragerwork, Aston Patterning, Craniosacral Therapy, Myofacial Release, Reflexology, Trigger Point Therapy, Baby Massage, Esalen Massage, Myotherapy, Rolfing, Vodder Lymph Drainage, The Benjamin System, Feldenkreis, Neuro Muscular Therapy, Sports Massage, Zero Balancing, Bindegewebsmassage, Hanna Somatics, On-Site Massage, Tellington Touch, Zone Therapy

---

Such a renaissance in the science and art of bodywork is unprecedented. There are several reasons for such a creative explosion of touch therapies in the twentieth century. I believe one of the most significant is the way in which the nurturing touch of massage was championed by the 'alternative' movement of the 1960s and 70s. The role of the Esalen Institute in Big Sur, California was seminal in this.

Esalen is considered by many to be the birthplace of the Human Potential Movement of those days and the role of massage was central to its culture (Calvert R. 2000). George Downing's "The Massage Book", portrayed Esalen style massage and became one of the 'bibles' of this movement. His drawings of naked hippies performing massage are now an icon to the age (Downing 1972). Later on, in the 80s, massage was championed as a genuinely holistic therapy that incorporated body, mind and spirit (Tappan F. 1980).

Another important reason for this transformation is that the demand for massage coincided with a phenomenal upsurge of popular interest in natural and more traditional healthcare modalities. As a result, alternative and complementary medicine has become one of the most rapidly developing sectors of the USA economy. Private and public sector massage training schools and independent practitioners have sprung up everywhere to meet this massive public demand. In a recent study of alternative and complementary medicine in the UK it was cautiously estimated that up to 15 million people have visited such practitioners. This constitutes 33 per cent of the population. In this same study, over 80 per cent of practitioners visited were found to be primarily using a touch therapy, and of these over 50 per cent were massage, aromatherapy or reflexology bodyworkers (Mills S. and Budd S 2000).

With this upsurge in popularity, practitioners and clients alike re-discovered what the ancient Greeks had known long ago: that massage helps the body to naturally restore balance and health. Herodicus, who was the teacher of Hippocrates in the 5th century BC, even claimed that he prolonged life with massage. Hippocrates himself was an ardent advocate of the therapeutic properties of massage, linking massage with diet and exercise as the three pillars of health and happiness (Graham 1884).

Modern stresses

It is also possible that modern-day massage has grown in stature as a therapy, in response to the stresses of a rapidly evolving society. Compared with previous centuries, society is now experiencing change at an alarmingly rapid rate. Change has become endemic. As a civilisation, managing the stresses involved in such changes has become one of our primary preoccupations. The arrival of the atomic bomb is just one dramatic example of the daily threat of annihilation that citizens across the globe now face. As a result of this and many other stresses, massage has evolved into a new and emergent therapy, which has also formed the basis of many new and creative bodywork and touch therapy modalities.

Reich

Massage in the nineteenth century was acknowledged as a powerful physical technique. In the twentieth century it also aligned itself with many of the psychological insights of the last hundred years since Freud. Much of this recognition came through the interest and explorations of Freud's gifted pupil, Wilhelm Reich (1897-1957). This has resulted in therapists and their clients claiming many powerful body–mind effects from massage as a therapy. Because many of our stresses also manifest themselves in structural imbalances, many of the new modalities of bodywork have emphasised deep tissue work and structural realignment. The amount of power and force needed to carry out these strong manipulations creates an additional strain on bodyworkers' thumbs and wrists.

Insurance

This enthusiastic bodywork has created additional problems for bodyworkers that were not present in the nineteenth century. Greene (1995) has pointed out that in America the massage profession has gained a modicum of acceptance from mainstream medical and allopathic doctors through insurance companies. This has resulted in massage therapists having to produce identifiable results to mainly structural problems. This has increased the pressure on practitioners to perform their deep structural techniques zealously – to the detriment of their hands.

Summary

In summary, then, it can now be argued that massage has evolved into a complete therapy in its own right. It appears that the healing potential of therapeutic massage and the benefits that touch can bring are becoming more evident to a modern society undergoing many stressful changes. In the twentieth century, massage and its many bodywork modalities most definitely became a therapy, whether 'structural' or 'body–mind'.

Massage, then, has changed considerably from Ling's use of a few techniques as an adjunct to a fitness program. It has changed, too, from the nineteenth-century use of techniques as part of a medical treatment. Modern-day massage practitioners are now using Ling's same 'occasional techniques' for the duration of the whole treatment session. This can mean anything from 50–90 minutes of continuous massage.

With all these changes to the profession of massage, it is no wonder that we are now discovering traditional techniques to have serious physical shortcomings for the practitioner. The injuries that are becoming common to practitioners are a direct consequence of these changes in the practice of massage over the last two centuries. Massage is now practiced in a totally different way and in a totally different setting from Ling's original Movement Cure.

As a profession, the implications for training schools are serious. To prepare our students for the new role that massage is now playing we must advocate new techniques that do not harm practitioners. Otherwise we run the risk of condemning our most successful practitioners to the most damaging injuries.

References

Adams A. "Degenerative Masseurs Syndrome" workshop presentation 2000

Benjamin P.J. "The Seeds of a Profession" The Massage Journal 41-47 1988

Calvert, R "Stars of the century" Massage Mag. Jan/Feb 2000

Cassar M.P. *The Massage Handbook* 1999

Downing G. *The Massage Book* 1972

Greene L. *Save Your Hands* 1995

Graham D. *A Treatise on Massage* New York Vail and Company 1885

Mackereth P. (Lecturer in Complementary studies, Salford University) - personal communication

Mills S. and Budd S. "Professional Organisation of Complementary and Alternative medicine in the UK 2000" A second report to the Dept of Health. University of Exeter. 2000

Porte D. R. 2000 (Professor of History of medicine, Welcome Trust, UK) - Personal communication

Pyves G. *NO-HANDS MASSAGE – Zero Strain Bodywork* Shi'Zen Publications 2000a.

Pyves G. *Massage Techniques are damaging Practitioners Hands* Shi'Zen Publications 2000b

Pyves G. *Massage History – From Technique to Therapy* Shi'Zen Publications 2000c

Pyves G. *No-Hands Massage – A new bodywork technology* Shi'Zen Publications 2000d.

Tappan F. "Healing Massage Techniques, Holistic, Classic and Emerging Methods" 1980 Appleton and Lange

Tracey C. "Massage Then and Now" Massage Winter 1992/3

Watson D. 2000 *An investigation into the links between massage practice and musculo-skeletal damage to the practitioner's hands and wrists* Shi'Zen publications Huddersfield

Van Der Why R.P. "Of what value is the Swedish Movement Cure?" Massage Therapy Journal Winter 1993)

Van der Why R.P. personal communication 2000

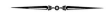

d. Application

"Ruaring Massage Brave" in the text was Ruari Martin and references to "Wise Woman Judy" were to Judy Midgley. Both are in regular Professional Development Groups with Gerry Pyves. Here is an account of their use of NO HANDS Chair Massage in a busy Yorkshire Hospital.

The use of muscle-based Chair Massage in a hospital setting

Judy Midgley (JM): The story begins at Clare Road, Halifax in April 2001, with Gerry Pyves teaching a NO HANDS Massage weekend. After years of practising conventional massage and suffering the effects, I was ready to give up altogether. I was inspired after seeing Gerry and his 'dancing troupe' at the ITEC Conference. I wanted to dance too. It was make-or-break time.

Ruari Martin (RM): This NO HANDS stuff was incredible and I wanted more. By lunchtime on Saturday we were signing up for the full practitioner course. There we were dancing and flying again for four more days. Judy and I had been talking about doing something together so doing the NO HANDS Chair Massage course was the next step to making this happen.

JM: Building on our NO HANDS training, we worked with a group of other experienced practitioners on the first NO HANDS Chair Massage course led by Gerry Pyves. I felt completely at ease with working with the chair. It was so right for me. I moved fluidly and easily from one move to the next. The zero-strain for me was even easier on the chair than the table. For the first time I knew that I could work all day with clients without tiring.

RM: Becoming a NO HANDS practitioner was unlocking my whole body for massage. NO HANDS Chair Massage liberated me again. It was so easy and so powerful and so simple to truly dance with my clients. At the end of that weekend I *was* the Dancing Bear!

JM: I had previously taught ITEC practitioner courses to a number of midwives and I also had nurses and doctors as clients in my practice. I knew from them how stressful their jobs were and how great was their need for massage. Some of the midwives had suggested I set up a practice at the hospital but I never felt it was an option until I had experienced the zero-strain approach of NO HANDS Chair Massage. I talked to Ruari. We both thought: "What a great idea! Let's give them what they want and need!". So I sent the proposal to a hospital Maternity Unit in West Yorkshire and waited.

RM: We heard nothing for the next 3-4 months. Actually we did hear on the grapevine about negative attitudes towards us and our work among certain managers at the hospital. So it came as a surprise when we had a phone call from a manager Midwife at the maternity unit. She loved our proposal - it helped that she was a trained massage practitioner herself - and we started planning the project together.

JM: There were many delays and obstacles but eventually, on June 21st 2002, a year after sending in the original proposal, we started at the hospital. It was a grand launch: Press, media, local NHS top-brass hierarchy. Arc-lights, flash bulbs, rubberneckers. Wine, buffet, speeches ... A real buzz about the place.

RM: And I remember thinking, as I sat waiting to be introduced before nearly a hundred expectant health professionals, "Aahh! What have I got myself into?" and, "Thank God we actually did that ten-minute run through half an hour ago". Anyway the launch was spectacular, a phenomenal success and established us immediately as potent and professional therapists.

We had spent a lot of time preparing for this project so that our delivery would be professional. Time was spent in adapting the Chair Massage to the on-site situation and doing extra training days with Gerry Pyves and with David Woodhouse. We had numerous discussions with staff at the unit. We both spent hours designing, researching, drafting and revising the project proposal. Before we'd even walked through their doors, we'd already done at least two weeks full-time work on the project!

JM: The key moment for me was when Ruari was demonstrating the Chair Massage on the Chief Exec's PA. I was commentating, and he had just finished working on her right arm/shoulder/neck complex and was moving to do the same at the other side. "Just look at her right shoulder", was all I needed to say, and they gasped as they noticed one shoulder a good six inches lower than the other. Dramatic and visible evidence that massage really works!

RM: Working with the nurses that summer was a joy. I felt at home doing my thing in an NHS inner-city hospital. The client group really appreciated my work and kept telling us what a big difference we were making. Plus I was getting paid properly for my valuable work. I tested the concept of zero-strain bodywork to the limit and it passed with flying colours. Working in this way was as healing for me as it was for them. I always left work feeling better than when I started.

JM: I had been away for a month without doing any massage. I was worried about coming back to doing the full day's massage with a possible fourteen clients! My back was already strained from an injury - two days before, I couldn't walk.

I was beginning to think that at 55 years old I should know better than to think I could keep up with Ruari, a young 'strap' of a man. I knew that it was important to keep fit and I had been exercising on holiday. I had decided to do Pilates to keep in shape, an exercise form which refers to the belly as the power house and follows yoga stretching and breathing techniques.

But my back was so bad that I couldn't move without pain, let alone exercise. I rang Ruari on the Sunday and told him I might not be able to do the massage. On Monday the back was manageable and Ruari was committed to other work. I felt really worried as I went into the hospital on Tuesday.

After the third treatment my back was really aching. I realised I wasn't using the correct postures. So I started moving from my belly as I had learnt with Gerry. Using my *Hara* as my powerhouse, I spread my legs wider so that they were fully supporting me. I focused on using my body weight throughout the massage ... using my breath as I danced round the client, back and forth, inhale, exhale, the massage became more like yoga ...

I could start to feel the benefits between massages and during the massage I was completely focussed on the client and on my dance with them. At the end of the day, after ten clients, I had no back pain at all, I felt completely free of aches and pains. The day's work had been a treatment for my back. 'Healer, heal thyself' indeed!

RM: We are involved with three separate departments at the hospital, continually refining the service we provide, learning all the time from our clients.

JM: It felt good to be working with Ruari after years of working on my own in private practice. I was ready to move on and move outwards and I loved working in the hospital environment. Caring for the carers means I have a chance to improve the way the NHS looks after its staff and, through this, improves its patient care.

When the staff returned to their work after the massage we heard how much more alert and relaxed they were. Members of staff regularly reported how changed their colleagues looked after receiving Chair Massage. There were so many anecdotal stories from staff:

One member of staff said that after her massage she felt so "chilled out" that she could go back to the ward and do anything she was asked to do without doing her normal thing of getting up tight!

Another member of staff reported how a shoulder pain disappeared and still hadn't come back six weeks later – a pain she had been plagued with for over three months!

These two responses show how both physiological and psychological aspects of people's working life are affected by Chair Massage.

From comments that staff were making, it was obvious to me that they were more relaxed and therefore able to enjoy their work. As a result of this they were also able to perform better.

There was also a knock-on effect on the other staff and the mood of the whole ward can change. The working environment became less stressful and therefore much more efficient. I believe that this can only benefit everyone - staff and patients alike.

RM: I feel strongly that I have arrived at the place where I want to work - in the public sector with dedicated people. I am bringing the power of healing touch right into the heart of ordinary people's everyday life. What greater satisfaction can there be for a bodyworker? And we haven't even touched the tip of the iceberg! Wherever we went in the hospital over the five months we were there, staff came up to us and demanded to know when this was going to become a permanent and regular service. If these were the results after only one or two sessions, then only the sky is the limit! We felt the most telling statistic was that only 13 per cent said they would prefer more money from their job! It is clear to us that people need so much more than just income from their work.

JM: So we are looking forward to the future. We intend to train as trainers with the NO HANDS Massage Company so that we can teach other practitioners how to do this effortless Chair Massage, and how to dance with their clients. We want every practitioner to learn how to enjoy a full day of massage and come out at the end of it feeling better than when they started. We hope to expand the business throughout the region and beyond. We shall improve working lives and – equally importantly – we will enjoy ourselves so much while doing it!

Evaluation

Here is an evaluation summary of our work in just one of the wards, where we massaged one day a week for two months. Most participants in this pilot project received only one or two massages each. Feedback was given only once by each participant immediately after the session. We wanted to ensure that negative comments could be made, so staff filled out their anonymous forms in private and stuffed them into an envelope themselves – an envelope full of other staff evaluations.

Evaluation Form

1. What did you get from your massage?

    (own words)

2. How satisfied are you with your massage

    10 - 9 – 8 – 7 – 6 – 5 – 4 – 3 – 2 – 1 - 0   (circle)

3. Have you had massage before?

    (Y/N)

4. If yes, how did it compare?

    Better   Just as Good   Not as Good   (circle)

5. Would you like a permanent Workplace Massage service for the unit?

    (Y/N)

6. If yes, would you like it to be

    Chair Massage   Table Massage   Either   (circle)

7. What exercise activities do you engage in during your leisure time?

    (own words)

8. Finally, please tell us which 3 things would improve your working life

    (own words)

    1   2   3

Summary of results Nov-Dec 2002

Trauma and Orthopaedic Unit

Sample: 54 members of staff completed the evaluation forms.

1. Benefits

More relaxed after the massage	78%
Invigorated, refreshed or energised	13%
Experienced a release of tension	13%

2. Satisfaction

Level 8 or above	90%
Level 10	48%

3. Previous massage

Previous experience of massage	50%

4. Comparisons (of above 50%)

Better or equally as good	78%

5. Permanent service?

Yes	100%

6. Chair or table?

Happy with the chair	89%

7. Exercise

No exercise	17%
Walking or swimming	76%

8. What would improve working life?

Less stress	42%
More staff	35%
More massage	31%
More time	24%
More money	13%

e. Chair Massage Research

"Petrissage Pete" in the text refers to Peter Mackereth and his hunting scout "Running Water" refers to Gwynneth Campbell.

"Chair Massage: A research and service evaluation"

Abstract

This paper addresses the issues relevant to considering conducting research with Chair Massage. Peter Mackereth, a PhD Student at the University of Manchester, examines the reasons for advocating research activities, possible methodologies and recommendations for further developing a research profile for NO HANDS Chair Massage. Gwynneth Campbell, who is lead practitioner for the Chair Massage for Carers Project, reports on the evaluation of services for carers and staff.

Introduction

Chair Massage typically involves a 15-minute treatment to the back, head, neck and hands. It does not require removal of clothing or use of oils. This makes it ideal for carers and patients able to receive massage in a seated position. Chair Massage has been available within the Christie Hospital Trust for three years, initially for staff but recently the service has been extended to carers and on a referral and assessment basis for in-patients. The lead practitioner on the Chair Massage for Carers Project is a qualified massage therapist and nurse, and is overseeing the project as part of his role. He has also taken part in a Chair Massage Research Project at the Touch Research Institutes (TRI), University of Miami's School of Medicine (Mackereth, 2001) and has completed Chair Massage training in the UK and US. The service currently provides Chair Massage on a referral basis for carers, defined as a partner, close friend or relative who is visiting daily and/or staying overnight at the hospital.

The importance of research and evaluation

The subjective experience of receiving massage usually informs members of the public in seeking and paying privately for further treatments and recommending a therapist to friends, family and work colleagues. There is also a growing interest in providing complementary therapy services within conventional health care settings, but service providers require evidence of benefit before considering employing therapists to treat patients (Cant and Sharma, 1996). The House of Lords Science and Technology Report (2000) reviewing complementary medicine has stressed the need for stronger evidence for the benefits of massage and other therapies popular with the public, and aims to improve professional regulation and awareness of potential risks and hazards. Many massage therapists and, indeed their teachers may not be fully informed of the research and evaluation work published and so may find it difficult to address the demand for the evidence, risks and costs from potential employers. Kahn (2001) has argued that massage schools have an important role in transforming massage into a research-conscious profession. It is important for practitioners to be active in accessing the literature, and where possible, formally evaluating their own practice. Aside from attending courses and conferences, clinical supervision for Chair Massage practitioners can also provide a space to review, inform and develop their practice (Mackereth 2002).

What constitutes acceptable evidence is debatable. Citing research findings may not be enough to convince potential funding agents. Providers may want to know the details. How many participants took part in the study? What type of research methods and outcome measures were used? Who conducted the study? Where was it published? There is also a hierarchy of evidence when it comes to reviewing published work. On the top of the list is the systematic review – the researcher here critically reviews existing research work and summarises the collective evidence (Ernst, 2001). Further down the list are trials, which randomise the participants and compare outcomes in groups including control subjects who do not receive the treatment under investigation. Some studies also use a placebo where both the research subjects and the researcher themselves do not know who is receiving the 'active' intervention – this is called the 'double-blind randomised controlled trial', and is particularly favoured in scientific research circles. In investigating massage it is not possible to use sham massage, given that subjects feel and experience the treatment. The following section is a review of recent studies evaluating Chair Massage that have been published by experienced researchers. Apart from the reference list at the end of this chapter, there is also a further reading list which contains important research texts relevant to complementary therapies.

Evidence and experience of using the massage chair

Chair Massage has been growing in popularity and can be seen being used in airports, public events, exhibitions and in health care settings. Its use in hospitals and hospices, for both patients and carers, is becoming more widely accepted with the increase of research and evaluation studies, clearly identifying the benefits of such interventions.

Recent research has reported that 15-minute sessions of Chair Massage reduce stress and enhance the electroencephalogram pattern of alertness in subjects. Field *et al* (1996) identified that a group of 26 subjects receiving Chair Massage twice a week for 5 weeks had more reduced anxiety levels, lowered cortisol readings, improved alertness and higher scores in computational tasks after treatment than the control group of 24 subjects. A key finding in a study by Cady and Jones (1997) was the significant lowering of both systolic and diastolic blood pressure of employees following a 15-minute on-site massage, although there was no control group for this study. Importantly for health-care workers, Field *et al* (1997) conducted a study in which hospital workers were given a 10-minute Chair Massage, after which decreases in anxiety, depression and fatigue were reported as well as increases in vigour. In another larger study by Hodge *et al* (2000), involving 100 health care workers, subjects were randomised into 2 groups, one group (n = 50) received 20 minutes of Chair Massage and the other, the control group, (n = 50) rested for an equal time period. Subjects who received Chair Massage exhibited decreases in blood-pressure recordings, anxiety and sleep disturbances, and improvements in well-being and emotional control. A service project providing massage to carers has been the subject of a published evaluation in the US (OHA and EWHA 1998). Thirteen caregivers were given an average of six massages, after which 85% reported emotional and physical stress level reduction, 77 per cent reported physical pain reduction and 54 per cent reported better patterns of sleep. In the UK a massage service for family members of patients receiving palliative care has been well evaluated by subjects participating in focus groups (Penson 1998).

This section has briefly reviewed a small number of published papers on Chair Massage. Attention has also been drawn to the work of Dr Tiffany Field whose team has conducted important and innovative research activities in this field. For further information, see the address list for details of the TRI website. It is important to acknowledge that there is a need for further work and in particular investigating the benefits of providing Chair Massage in hospital settings. Box 1 is a suggested list of areas for further research work.

Implementation of the Chair Massage for Carers project at Christie Hospital

Three portable, ergonomically designed padded massage chairs have been purchased as a result of a successful bid to charitable funds. The service currently provides Chair Massage on a referral basis for carers; defined as a partner, close friend or relative. The portability of the chairs enables the therapists to deliver the treatment to the relatives wherever they are in the hospital (by the bedside, dayrooms or out in the gardens). This innovative project has already been the subject of a recent published paper (Mackereth and Campbell 2002).

Rationale for the innovation

The complementary service was initially established for patients; however, as the service developed, staff frequently asked therapists to treat stressed/distressed relatives. The innovative idea to provide a Chair Massage service was proposed by the Complementary Therapy Coordinator and supported by the Complementary Therapy Committee. An important goal for the Trust is to fulfil the recommendations of the Cancer Plan (DoH 2000) to evaluate complementary therapies not only for patients, but also for carers. Recent records indicate that referrals are increasing to in excess of ten per week for this intervention.

Preparation of practitioners

An intensive two-day Chair Massage course has been designed specifically for massage therapists wishing to expand their complementary therapy skills in palliative care. Adapting treatments to suit individuals' needs, whether they be a patients or carers, is of paramount importance, and the training includes ways of adapting Chair Massage for people who are ill or distressed. (For guidance on considering offering Chair Massage, see Boxes 2 and 3.)

At present there are 6 massage therapists working part-time at Christie Hospital, all of whom have successfully completed the course. The training is now available nationally and has generated income for the pilot project.

Evaluation strategy

Documentation has been prepared with the guidance of the Audit Department to gather data about all the access and provision of complementary therapy interventions. Data is collected for the purpose of evaluation from this treatment sheet. Feedback following the treatment is obtained using a 'feel-good thermometer', a visual analogue scale used to evaluate well-being pre- and post- a therapeutic intervention (Field 2000). It is a way of recording the subjective feel-good factor on a scale of 0–10 (0 being "not feeling good at all" and 10 being "the best I've ever felt") (Field 2000). Those receiving treatment also have a chance to say how they feel afterwards. The number of treatments received is also noted, as is how they heard of the service and who referred them, ranging from self-referral, nursing staff or seeing notices around the hospital, to the complementary therapists themselves passing through the wards. Other details such as the relationship to the patient are recorded. For this evaluation study it did not seem appropriate to measure blood pressure, pulse rate or other physical reactions that are often associated with research into evidence for the use of complementary therapies, as we are dealing with people who are often in a very vulnerable state. This is first and foremost a real life easing of pain and discomfort and not primarily a research study. Those receiving a treatment are asked if they mind helping the evaluation by completing the 'feel-good thermometer', which is on the back of the consultation sheet, where routine health questions appear which would be asked prior to any intervention. The project is ongoing so final conclusions cannot be reached. From the early data there is growing evidence that the service is having a big impact, both in terms of popularity and in reported benefits (see Box 4).

Box 4: Reported benefits of Chair Massage

- Relaxation
- Time for attention and support
- Supported posture
- Assistance with pain and muscular stiffness
- Reduced anxiety
- Improvement in mood
- Revitalisation and refreshment

Mackereth and Campbell (2002)

Initial and potential impact on the Trust and Rehabilitation Service

Since the project began on 26 June 2002 we have so far completed over 110 treatments. Initial trends indicate that requests for the service are spreading throughout the hospital, and are especially popular with parents in the Young Oncology Unit (30 per cent of total treatments), all of whom report considerable increase in well-being and relaxation. We feel that this innovative service is already proving popular and will contribute towards the welfare of patients' relatives, one of the stated aims of the NHS Plan (DoH, 2000).

From the first 110 recipients of Chair Massage, no one has reported feeling worse than before the treatment, and almost all reported increases of between 2 and 5 degrees on the 'thermometer', with 5 reporting 9 or 10 degrees' difference.

This early data has identified 20 per cent reporting a 0–2 increase in feelings of well-being, 60 per cent showing increases ranging from 3– 5. 20 per cent reported 6–10 degrees of increase. Two carers reported the maximum increase (10), one of whom appears in the case study below.

Case Study 1

A patient's partner had been sleeping with considerable discomfort in a chair beside the patient's bed for two weeks. He was afraid to leave in case his partner's condition deteriorated. The referral for Chair Massage was made by one of the ward staff. The carer reported feeling tense and exhausted prior to the massage. Their response on the 'feel-good thermometer' following the 15-minute treatment went from 0 to 10. The carer reported relaxing completely during the treatment and their muscle tension easing. After resting for a few moments he returned to his vigil noticeably refreshed. The next day a member of the nursing team stopped to thank the practitioner, and to report that the patient had died peacefully with their carer awake and calmly present at the bedside.

Over two-thirds of the participants were women, most being parents of young people on the Young Oncology Unit. About two-thirds of those participating reported musculo-skeletal problems prior to treatment. Afterwards people said they felt more relaxed, more mobile, looser and refreshed, the vast majority using the words ' relaxed' or 'very relaxed' to describe how they felt after the Chair Massage. Obviously there could be some element of wishing to please the therapist, which maybe has some 'halo' affect on how the treatment is viewed. To limit this we asked carers to fill in the 'thermometer' themselves, without the therapist seeing. The next stage in the project is to employ an independent interviewer who we hope will be able to ascertain more impartial feedback. A report will be prepared on this first stage of the project and a presentation made to the Complementary Therapy Committee, who will review it and then advise on its further development.

Chair massage for staff and volunteers

A Chair Massage service has been available to staff for three years, and has recently been part-funded by staff amenities fund, so can be accessed at a discounted rate via the Occupational Health Department. In addition, staff returning to work after illness may be entitled to free vouchers for up to three Chair Massage or other complementary therapy sessions. This service is in constant demand, and feedback has been positive. In a work setting, the advantage of receiving massage without getting the hair or clothes oily remains high, and contributes greatly to its popularity. The feeling of relaxation gained in just a few minutes is very important.

Bio-dots

At a well-being day for hospital staff, the effect of Chair Massage was recorded by using bio-dots. These are manufactured in the USA and can be obtained from 'Stresswise' in the UK (see address list). One can be placed on the skin over a blood vessel at the wrist or back of the hand, and it changes colour according to a chart, which accompanies the biodots. A note is made of the colour before and after treatments, and this can show a change in the blood flow and, accordingly, the degree of relaxation. In almost every case the results showed some measurable amount of relaxation. This emphasises that it is not just the muscles that are being relaxed by massage, but it also favourably affects circulation. An evaluation of the well-being event was conducted and feedback from participants requested. Over 160 members of staff attended the day and the positive feedback, including specific comments on the benefits of Chair Massage, has helped in securing funds to develop complementary therapy services for staff. This provision is now also the subject of an ongoing service evaluation.

Conclusion – where to from here?

The rise in the popularity of Chair Massage and subsequent developments in its delivery, from using the 'NO HANDS' approach to adapting treatments to suit cancer patients, their carers and hospital staff, demonstrates that there is a growing demand for clothed, seated and safe forms of short massage treatments. Our hospital-based Chair Massage projects have kick-started interest in receiving massage from people who may not ordinarily seek out therapeutic massage. We have also noticed frequently the therapeutic value to patients of watching a close friend/relative receive a Chair Massage. Maybe this observation indicates that there are benefits of seeing your anxious and stressed relative let go and receive nurturing at a time when it is hard for you to hold them (see Case Studies 1 and 2). It is also important to acknowledge that finding helpful intervention to support both patient and their carers can also have benefits for clinical staff, who at times may feel at a loss in providing support. These considerations provide added reasons for extending and researching the service.

Case Study 2

The intervention of Chair Massage on one occasion in a hospital room to an apparently highly anxious partner of an ill patient, transformed the scene from one of fluster and anxiety to one of peace and tranquillity, leaving both the patient and relative in a state of deep relaxation.

This paper has overviewed the research evidence for Chair Massage and reported on ongoing service evaluation projects being conducted within a hospital setting. The authors are happy to receive enquiries from practitioners wishing to hear more about our work and can be contacted through Christie Hospital.

Peter A Mackereth MA RGN RNT Dip Reflex Adv Reflex (Level 3) ABMT Practitioner and Lecturer in Complementary Therapies, Christie Cancer Hospital Manchester and Salford University.

Gwynneth Campbell BA(Hons) PGCE Dip Th Mass (APNT) MIPTI, NO HANDS Massage Practitioner and Research Assistant, Christie Hospital Manchester

References

Cady S.H. and Jones G.E. (1997) "Massage therapy as a workplace intervention for reduction of stress". Perceptual and Motor Skills. 84(1): 157-158.

Cant S. and Sharma U. (1996) "Professionalisation of complementary medicine in the United Kingdom". Complementary Therapies in Medicine 4, 157-162.

DoH (2000) The NHS Cancer Plan. Department of Health HMSO. London

Ernst E. (2001) "Evidence-based massage therapy: a contradiction in terms". In: Rich G.J. (Eds) *Massage Therapy: the evidence for practice*. Harcourt Brace. London.

Field T. (2000) *Touch Therapy*. Harcourt Press London

Field T., Ironson G., Scafidid F., Nawrocki T., Goncalves A., Burman I., Pickens J., Fox N., Schanberg S. and Kuhn C. (1996) "Massage therapy reduces anxiety and enhances EEG pattern of alertness and maths computations". International Journal of Neurosciences 86(3-4): 197-205.

Field T. Quintino O. Henteleff Wells-Keife L. and Delvecchio-Feinberg G. (1997) "Job stress-reduction therapies". Alternative Therapies in Health and Medicine 3(4): 54-56.

Hodge M., Robinson C. and Boehmer Klein S, (2000) "Employee outcomes following work-site acupressure and massage". Massage Therapy Journal 39(3):48-64.

House of Lords Select Committtee on Science and Technology Sixth Report (2000) Complementary and Alternative Medicine. London: Stationery Office.

Kahn J. (2001) "Research Matters". Massage Magazine. Issue 92 July/August

Mackereth P. (2000) "Tough places to be tender: contracting for happy or 'good enough' endings in therapeutic massage/bodywork?" Complementary Therapies in Nursing and Midwifery. 6: 111-115.

Mackereth P. (2001) Touch Research Institutes; an interview with Dr Tiffany Field. Complementary Therapies in Nursing and Midwifery 7, 84-89.

Mackereth P. (2002) "Biodynamic massage and research". Journal of the Association of Holistic Biodynamic Massage Therapists. Winter/Spring Edition

Mackereth P, and Campbell G. (2002) "Chair Massage: attention and touch in 15 minutes". Palliative and Cancer Matters Issue 25: 2 and 6.

Oregon Hospice Association and East-West College of Healing Arts (1998) "Massage as a respite intervention for primary caregivers". American Journal of Hospice and Palliative Care Jan/Feb: 43-47

Penson J. (1998) "Complementary therapies: making a difference in palliative care Complementary Therapies in Nursing and Midwifery" 4(3): 77 – 81

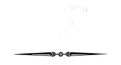

Further reading

Ferrell-Torry A.T., Glick O.J. (1993) "The use of therapeutic massage as a nursing intervention to modify anxiety and the perception of cancer pain". Cancer Nursing 16:93-101.

Foundation for Integrated Medicine (1997) "Integrated healthcare: a way forward for the next five years?" London: FIM

Graham L., Goldstone L., Eijundu A., Baker J. and Asiedu-Addo E. (1998) "Penetration of complementary therapies into NHS trust and private hospital practice". Complementary Therapies in Nursing and Midwifery 4(6):160-165.

Mitchell A. Cormack M. (1998) "The Therapeutic Relationship in Complementary Health Care". Churchill Livingstone London

Montbriand M. J. (1998) "Abandoning biomedicine for alternative therapies: oncology patients' stories". Cancer Nursing 21(1): 36-45

Spencer J. W. and Jacobs J. J. (1999) *Complementary/alternative medicine: an evidence-based approach.* Mosby London.

Watson D. (2000) *An investigation into the links between massage practice and musculoskeletal damage to the practitioner's hands and wrists.* Shi'Zen Publications Huddersfield

Vickers A. (1995) "A basic introduction to medical research. Part 3: what can the practitioner do?" Complementary Therapies in Nursing and Midwifery. 1,143-147.

Suggested further reading

The Lone Ranger still maintains that there is only one bodywork book really worth reading, and that is Don McFarland's *Body Secrets.* (Healing Arts Press) ISBN 0-944504-00-0. If you haven't read this then you have such a treat in store! It is a gem.

The first book of the NOHANDS trilogy *The Principles and Practice of NO HANDS Massage* (Shi'Zen Publications) ISBN 0-9539074-0-6 provides a vital support to this book.

Another important book for understanding the extent of the injury problem is Lauriann Greene's *Save Your Hands* (Gilded Age Press) ISBN 0-9679549-0-8

Regarding historical material a wonderful book is Kurre Ostrom's *Massage and the original Swedish movements* (Octagon Press) ISBN 0-9518025-0-X

An excellent and clear description of meridian-based Chair Massage can be found in Patricia Abercromby and Davina Thomson's *Seated Acupressure Massage* (Corpus Publishing) ISBN 1-903333-01-6

A great contribution to Chair Massage literature can be found in Shogo's Mochizuchi's *Japanese Chair-Massage Techniques* ISBN 1-57615-040-2 and some excellent hand-protection exercises can be found in his highly informative *Hand Maintenance Guide* ISBN 1-57615-075-5 (Kotobuchi publications, Colorado)

For all wisdom and expert information about massage we strongly recommend your belly, because inside your belly is all the bodywork wisdom in the world! And for anything else, just get really busy and develop that attunement.

All these books can be located through the NO HANDS web site:

www.nohandsmassage.com

Useful addresses and web sites

For the work of the NO HANDS Massage Company, including their muscle-based Chair Massage trainings:

PO BOX 57, Hebden Bridge, W. Yorks HX7 6WW

Tel: 0870-24-30-876

www.nohandsmassage.com

enquiries@nohandsmassage.com

For the work of The Academy of On-Site Massage, including their highly professional zero-strain meridian-based Chair Massage training:

Avon Road, Charfield, Wootton-under-Edge, Gloucestershire GL12 8TT

Tel: 01454-269269

www.aosm.co.uk

all@aosm.co.uk

Going to the source, the web site of the founder of Chair Massage is well worth a visit. David Palmer's site gives much valuable information about his work and his organisation.

www.touchpro.org

In the UK, another useful Chair Massage contact is the Seated Acupressure Massage Training School,

www.acupressure-training.co.uk

A great bodywork site for much additional historical material including many relevant books is:

www.massagemag.com

To contact Ruari Martin and Judy Midgely and their Workplace Massage Company, go to:

www.workplace-massage.co.uk

To contact Peter Mackereth and Gwynneth Campbell write or ring:

c/o The Rehabilitation Unit Christie Hospital, Wilmslow Rd., Manchester M20 4BX

Tel: 0161 446 3795

Dr Tiffany Field's research work is located at the Touch Research Institute:

www.miami.edu/touch-research/triresearch.htm

To get hold of the fascinating 'Biodots', contact:

'Stresswise', PO Box 5, Congleton, Cheshire CW 1XE